A Practical Guide to
HIP SURGERY

From
Pre-Op to Recovery

M. E. HECHT, M.D.

SUNRISE
River Press

Sunrise River Press
39966 Grand Avenue
North Branch, MN 55056
Phone: 651-277-1400 or 800-895-4585
Fax: 651-277-1203
www.sunriseriverpress.com

Edit by Karin Craig
Layout by Monica Seiberlich
Illustrations by D. M. Smith

ISBN 978-1-934716-12-0
Item No. SRP612

Library of Congress Cataloging-in-Publication Data

Hecht, M. E.
  A practical guide to hip surgery : from pre-op to recovery / by M. E. Hecht.
    p. cm.
  ISBN 978-1-934716-12-0
  1. Hip joint--Surgery--Popular works. I. Title.
  RD549.H43 2011
  617.5'81059--dc22
                              2010016564

Printed in USA
10 9 8 7 6 5 4 3 2 1

Contents

Dedication

To the moon, sun, and stars in my life. But most especially to "D," without whom this *vade mecum* would not have been possible. Especial thanks to my invaluable editor, Karin Craig.

Foreword by Dr. Gerald Imber

An astounding 450,000 hip replacements are performed annually in the United States. Even more astounding is the pervasive ignorance surrounding this procedure. For most patients hip replacement will offer a "gift of mobility," but they cannot afford to enter into this miraculous surgery without Dr. Mary Ellen Hecht's insightful *A Practical Guide to Hip Surgery*.

This unique book comes at the problem from both sides. For not only is Dr. Hecht an expert orthopedic surgeon and teacher, she is also a hip replacement patient. Dr. Hecht provides the patient with a step-by-step on how to prepare for surgery, recovery, and what to expect after surgery. The *Guide* will help prospective patients understand and prepare for their surgery, and may well be the most comprehensive book of its kind.

Dr. Hecht has spent a career as an educator of doctors and patients alike, and with this book will become your trusted advisor as you face the prospect of hip surgery.

> *Dr. Imber is an internationally known surgeon. In addition to his private clinic in Manhattan, he is on the staff of the New York–Presbyterian Hospital, and the Weill Cornell Medical College in Qatar. He has written numerous scientific papers and several books, and lectured widely. He is a graduate of State University of New York Downstate Medical Center.*

This is a book about Total Hip Replacement (THR) and Hip Resurfacing (Resurf) surgery. It is also a self-help manual for those of you who are faced with arthritis of the hip and who may, at this moment, be booked or even hospital-bound for surgery.

I am an orthopedic surgeon whose practice was based in New York City. I've performed many THRs on patients referred to me by other doctors, as well as on patients in my own orthopedic practice. After many years of performing hip surgeries as a surgeon, I suddenly found myself in need of having both of my own hips replaced. And so, you see, I've been both *next to* and *on* the table; I am uniquely familiar with THR, from the perspectives of both a surgeon and a patient.

This book contains useful information about the risks and benefits of THR and Resurf surgery, about hospitals and doctors, and about pre-and post-operative happenings. For you who will face this surgery in the foreseeable future, it is my hope to make the prospect clearer, less daunting, and just possibly a more controllable experience.

I have always taught my orthopedic residents and medical students that if they really grasp a complicated medical concept, no matter how serious, they should discuss it with patients in straightforward terms. They need to be able to convey the heart of the matter in words that avoid convolution and "doctor-speak," Latinized multi-syllabic terms.

"Medicalese" is for medical conferences, not for patients who need surgery. Its use constitutes unnecessary cruelty on the part of the one in control of the patient/doctor dialogue, the one in charge of an impending surgical situation.

Having said that, I must use a Latin phrase to describe the essence of this book; the phrase is *vade mecum*, literally translates to "go with me." The ancient Romans used *vade mecum* to mean the indispensable traveler's kit that they kept with them everywhere and always. Thus, I hope you pack along this companion book when you leave for the hospital and keep it with you during your hip replacement or resurfacing experience and recovery.

In the early twentieth century, a brilliant young German poet, who unfortunately died during World War I, said, speaking of his craft, "a real poet doesn't say the sky is azure, he says the sky is blue." And so I hope you find this *vade mecum* for your forthcoming hip replacement is filled with blueness and strictly avoids the azure.

How to Use this Handbook

You will find as you read through this book that I have, as a surgeon, a fundamental belief in my patient's participation in the surgical process to the fullest extent possible. As a surgeon I always looked for a "junior partner" from my patients. The reason was that I wanted them to try for the fullest understanding of how we would get from A to Z, or from medical problem to solution. Such a "junior partner" makes a real difference in how things actually go from disability to recovery.

If I can answer patient questions, concerns, and worries as they come up, putting both my patient and me on the "same page," we both benefit. Therefore, at the end of each chapter, you will find *Your Space*. You can use this area to make notes and jot down questions for your doctor.

Based on the questions my patients have asked me over the years, I've suggested a few focus topics. This list of topics is by no means complete, and they may not fit you precisely, but they can serve as starting points.

I hope that as you go through the process of a THR or Resurf you won't settle for being a passive participant in what your body is about to undergo. If you make time to think about some of the suggestions on these pages, several things may happen:

1. You won't forget things you really wanted to ask about.
2. You will have a kind of journal preserving where you've been and how you got from there to recovery.
3. You'll never have the excuse, when asked about it by someone near and dear, "Well, I know I went through it, but I don't remember the details."
4. The notes, questions, and phenomena you record will convert you into a positive "active participant" and recorder of what will be, after all, a major happening in your life.

So give it a whirl. You may find you like it.

P.S. Go to Chapter Sixteen for essential checklists as soon as you start your own hip journey. And use it liberally and often throughout your Hip Journey.

Chapter One

My Story

On a spring day in New York City, I was wheeled into the operating room at Cabrini Hospital to have both of my hips replaced. The amount and kind of equipment I saw around me was massive. Technicians and operating room (O.R.) nurses were organizing and laying out the instruments that my orthopedic surgeon and his assistants would need during the procedure. The anesthesiologist was readying her medications. The room was filled with efficiency and purpose. Voices were more or less quiet. But over all of this I could distinctly hear the clink of equipment being handled and placed and surgical "spacesuits" being put on, connected, and tested.

As a surgeon, I understood and approved of the efficiency and purpose in the room. As a surgical patient, lying flat on my back on the operating table, I could only wait and watch patiently—as you will. I was an unusual patient in that I could hardly wait for the surgery to begin. But yet, I was the usual patient in that I would not settle for an existence of constant pain, life dependent on canes or crutches, even wheelchair bound, God forbid, for the rest of my life.

During my time waiting on the table for surgery to begin, my mind went to others lying in these same circumstances who would likely be fearful, or doubtful, or even just plain panicky.

I could understand that they might dread the operation to come, that they might question the wisdom of their decision and worry about their post-operative condition or even their survival—none of these being unreasonable or outrageous thoughts for a patient to have at this moment.

Then I remembered all the planning and problems—the thoughts and feelings that had landed me in this surgical room. I smiled to myself and thought, all things being equal and all systems go, I would like to share my experience with those who in the upcoming years would be going into similar operating rooms under similar conditions.

Then the thought of a *vade mecum* came to me and I became determined to write a companion book for fellow THR "havers." I knew the procedure like the back of my hand. I had, after all, performed the same operation many times, on many patients before I retired from the active practice of orthopedic surgery. As a matter of fact, I'd even done them in the same hospital and in the same operating room.

My surgeon, Dr. Richard Pearl, was one of my old orthopedic residents whom I'd "taken through" his first hip replacement. When I decided to go forward with the surgery, Dr. Pearl confessed that he was a little nervous working on me. I knew what he meant; in the role of patient, doctors are often wiseacres—difficult, abrasive, and intrusive in their own care. All of us as surgeons have had to deal with this situation at least once. Deciding to be part of the solution, not the problem, I promised Dr. Pearl that I would be "patient," and he could be "doctor" all the way—a decision I never regretted.

And so this book was born, in the immediacy of my surgery, and with the thought that I was uniquely suited to filling in the blanks for potential hip-replacement candidates. After all, I had years both doing and teaching the procedure and at this moment I was about to be a THR recipient.

Now that I've been the one *on*—rather than *next to*—the operating table, looking up at the super-bright lights of the operating room, the masked faces of the surgeon and technicians, the quantity of instruments laid out to be used during the procedure, I know how you may feel as you face hip surgery. Looking back, one additional talisman I can offer you is to remember the ability of your surgeon, and trust in his or her judgment training, experience, and even equipment.

Perhaps a brief calendar of how and why I arrived at the operating room at Cabrini Hospital would be helpful for purposes of comparison, and because the history is far from unusual.

Calendar of Events Leading to Surgery

At 70 years of age I was almost the exact median age for a THR. Four years earlier, my initial symptoms actually began in my *knees*, with marked pain and swelling, aggravated by walking. I had no hip pain, none at all. However, I noticed when I looked in the mirror that I was bent forward at the hip when walking or even standing—which I thought related to sparing my knees.

As the pain in my knees worsened, I began to limit the surgeries I performed to those that could be done sitting down. Many were performed as same-day surgery, so there were no hospital rounds to make. I also stopped taking emergency room calls, but still managed to do consulting in orthopedics.

My lab workups were all normal values except for a slightly high erythrocyte sedimentation rate (ESR), which is a non-specific blood test that comes back elevated if there is any kind of inflammation or even infection of the body. No diabetes. No rheumatoid factors, no abnormal hormones. My calcium levels were great. I ran through all the standard oral medications, both non-steroidal (e.g., ibuprofen, feldene, voltarin, relafen, etc.) and steroidal (prednisone and others) without help. I also injected my own knees several times with cortisone, with little relief.

Finally, I had my knees x-rayed, which showed minimal signs of wear and tear. Nothing commensurate with the pain and stiffness I was experiencing. Mind you, it was all I could do to walk a city block—about one-tenth of a mile.

Eventually I had to throw in the towel and quit my practice. My knees simply wouldn't let me do daily rounds or care properly for my patients. At 66, with all my skills and experience intact, I was forced to retire from active practice.

What Then?

I moved to Paris and went back to an old love—writing. My physical activities became lamentably limited. Why even try to exercise when the only result was to subject myself to pain. Sure, I could swim, and I felt terrific when I was in the water, but the horror of getting in and out of the pool via ladders! Even changing in and out of a bathing suit had become a problem. Forget about getting stockings on by myself! I went to some concerts and plays, but less and less often as they became more difficult to handle (*How far from the car to the theater entrance? How long were the aisles, where was my seat in a row? How many steps or escalators did I need to manage?*).

In common with many people, I adore movies—but the consideration of getting into and out of the crimped motorized vehicles which are called New York City cabs—much less moving about in Paris—forget it!

My home video bill grew by leaps and bounds. Forced to sit much of the time, and with eating an unalloyed pleasure, I started to gain quantities of weight. My friends still loved me, but they winced as they watched me crawl by with the help of two canes, canted forward at 30 degrees, and looking more like a beached crab than a human being.

You may remember the wonderful line of Tevya in *Fiddler on the Roof,* "Because you've had a bad day, should I suffer?" I've always been something of a stoic, and have always agreed with Tevya when it came to complaints. So I kept still about my pain and discouragement. But when alone at night, sometimes I did break down and weep. I saw no answers, and nowhere to go but down.

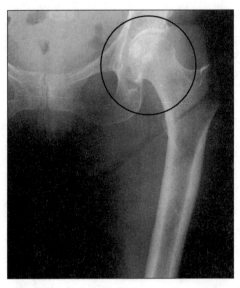

This is a nearly normal hip. The femoral head (ball) is smooth and symmetrical. The acetabulum (socket) is clear. Joint space is maintained, with possible loose body in the joint, and mild breaking (osteophyte formation) at the top of the acetabulum.

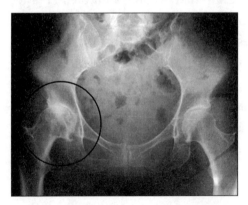

On the left is shown advanced arthritis. The femoral head is mis-shapened and the joint space is narrowed and irregular. On the right is a nearly normal hip.

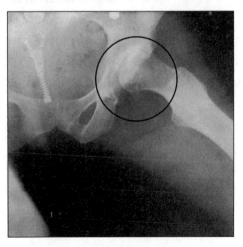

This x-ray shows marked arthritis. Both ball and socket show irregular shape. Osteophytes are clearly shown at the femoral head. Loose body is evident.

As time passed pain, stiffness, and disability ruled my world. A quarter of a city block was out of the question; my waking hours were spent in a chair in front of the computer. I was taking Tylenol #4 (containing 60 mg of codeine) for pain several times a day, and I dreaded the nighttime. Intense knee pain woke me in bed, if I turned the wrong way. At the absolute best, sleep was what has been nicely described as fitful. We all know what kind of day follows a sleepless night, and a series of sleepless nights makes dragons out of the most cheerful of us. Being an orthopedic surgeon, *I knew* I was doing all that could be done for my knees, using the latest medications. The future looked—no fooling—bleak.

Finally, I began to feel mild pain in my hips too. Pain that I was sure was secondary compensation for my knee problems. At the insistence of a good friend, I went to see a rheumatologist who insisted on taking x-rays of my *hips*. I explained with a little condescension that it was my *knees* that had brought me to his office, but it was his office and his call so I went off to have my hips x-rayed, laughing to myself at his denseness.

Imagine my embarrassment, much less horror, when he put my hip films up on the view box. There I saw not one, but two, far-gone arthritic hips. It was hard to decide which side was worse. Both were distorted, narrowed, and over-calcified.

It doesn't take much to see the difference between a healthy versus needful ball-and-socket hip joint—one has only to look at the disappearing joint space and the incongruity between surfaces. The more you use a hip joint in this unsymmetrical state, the worse it becomes, and the more you need to think about having surgery.

Finally meeting his eyes, I said, "So, no need for further discussion, doctor. THRs are needed, and not one, but two." To his eternal credit, as there is still much of the Hatfield/McCoy-type disagreement between internists and surgeons with respect to the best solutions to medical problems, he replied simply, "I agree." Right then and there I had a second surgical opinion, and afterward was off to see Dr. Pearl.

Later it dawned on me that many of my patients had complained more of knee pain than of hip pain. But I hadn't grasped before this that a thoroughly arthritic hip could be silent, a lessoned learned even after years of practice. Now I'm not at all sure this is an atypical presentation of the problem. It has to do with what is called referred pain, where nerve conduction (a complicated system at best) fools us about just where the source of the pain lies. In effect, your body scams you by saying it's your knee that's in trouble, when in fact it's your hip.

For me at this point, despite the fact that total hip replacements are classified as "elective," it was not an adjective that could reasonably be applied. It was only a matter of when, where, and who.

I had arrived at the point where my regular internist wanted to go over my personal risks and benefits vis-à-vis the surgery. Every patient's risks are a bit different.

My medical problems, not uncommon ones, were that I was overweight and struggling with high blood pressure, both the result of my completely sedentary lifestyle for the past two years.

As a surgeon, I knew that although these were risk factors, they were not inherently major deterrents to surgery. Other THR candidates have far more serious problems that need to be minimized, or at least stabilized, before surgery should be considered; namely hormonal, cardiac, or circulatory, to name a few. Of course, when all is said and done, a patient's internist or medical doctor must "clear" his patient for surgery and agree that all risks considered, the surgery should go forward.

It was November when I saw the rheumatologist. After that visit I lost more than 60 pounds by dieting. I also did chair-type exercises to strengthen my legs and some lap swimming for general conditioning. Not perfect pre-op conditioning, but certainly better than none. And, come May, I ventured into Cabrini Hospital and onto the operating room table.

How Do You Know It's Your Hips?

C onsider how I discovered I needed hip surgery. You will most likely identify with one or more of these phenomena:

- Gait change—even subtle unevenness or favoring of one leg or the other.
- Knee pain with or without swelling, and even possible buckling.
- Back pain, especially if it has arrived after a gait change or knee pain. X-rays of the spine do not show a clear reason for your back pain.
- Stiffness of hip joint, resulting in such things as trouble getting up stairs, even one flight; difficulty getting into and out of cars; trouble rising from a chair, especially low ones; limping in the morning or after sitting for a while; and thinking twice about how far it may be to get to anywhere.
- Groin or buttock pain.
- A change in posture, often noted first by a friend or partner.

In discussing the problem, which is now identified as a hip problem, your doctor may well use the word osteoarthritis. Lots of people, including medical experts, physical therapists, etc., have described various kinds of arthritis. Here is my version, so you know where your hip fits in.

"Arthritis" itself is a catchall phrase meaning an inflammation or breakdown of a joint—and that's all it means. It can affect any joint of the body, from toes to spine. It always implies some degree of pain, some degree of limitation of range of motion (stiffness), and some degree of objective evidence, usually seen as bony changes and/or excessive joint fluid on an x-ray. It's also what folks mean when they use the term "rheumatism."

Osteoarthritis

The most common form of arthritis is osteoarthritis—the arthritis associated with advancing age. It is reliably estimated that some 45 million people suffer from osteoarthritis in this country. That's 50 to 60 percent of all people over 70 years of age. And by the year 2030, approximately 70 million people age 65 and over will be identified as having osteoarthritis with hips, knees, shoulders, and spine being the most common sites.

We used to think this was simply a matter of wear and tear until we realized that life span alone (a long period of wear and tear) didn't produce osteoarthritis in everyone. Now we know it probably starts as a congenital or genetic condition—isn't everything these days! In other words, you're born with a subtly incongruous hip anatomy, which poses no trouble at all for a number of years of activity, but in time, the hip finally wears out and becomes arthritic.

The other genetic theory is that you're born with an imbalance in the enzymes of the cartilage or lining of the hip joint, causing it to gradually break down, ending in the condition we recognize as arthritis. That is not to say that wear and tear or injuries don't aid and abet. They certainly do. Sometimes a severe hip fracture or dislocation can result in arthritis. But that's not the usual culprit.

Think of family histories, and likely you will find that osteoarthritis tends to "run in families." The unvarnished truth is that it doesn't matter whether you're a sedentary bookworm or a gung-ho jock, a marathoner or a couch potato; if your hip anatomy is off, you can't prevent or avoid it. After a certain number of years, usually 60 plus, the small anatomical anomalies of your hip degenerate into osteoarthritis.

If osteoarthritis remains a mild-to-moderate condition, it may respond to anti-inflammatory medication (Motrin, Naprosyn, ibuprofen, or the like) and gentle exercise. If not, you're looking at the probability sooner or later of a THR or possibly a Resurf.

There are a few additional causes, but they are rare. Osteoarthritis is the common garden variety of hip joint arthritis. On x-ray, the hip joint is narrowed and shows irregularity, often losing much of its normal congruence. Its symptoms include pain, stiffness, and occasionally sound effects (creaking or cracking).

As the hip joint continues to lose its normal smooth bearing cartilage (bone cover), bone grates on bone.

Other Causes of Hip Arthritis

Are there other conditions that can lead to hip arthritis? Yes, but they represent only about 10 to 12 percent of cases. They're usually associated with medical conditions or systemic problems:
- Traumatic Arthritis.
- Rheumatoid Arthritis, Lupus, and other autoimmune diseases.
- Hematological problems—e.g., sickle cell disease, and even sickle cell trait.
- Gout.

- Hypothyroidism.
- Mild to severe congenital hip malformation/incongruity present at birth—it doesn't seem critical whether they're diagnosed and treated or not.
- Severe trauma to the hip (fractures and dislocations).
- Alcoholism.
- Overuse of steroids (the jury is still out on androgens—the muscle-builders too often used by "athletes"—but the possibility is far from remote).

Traumatic Arthritis

The second most common form of arthritis is called traumatic arthritis, and it acts absolutely the same. The pain experienced is just as common. Traumatic arthritis can be produced by an unsuspected onset; a severe tumble or motor vehicle accident in the past may show up over the years as arthritis, or it may also come from a frank fracture or dislocation, even perfectly treated at the time of incident. Then too at an early age, the abuse of repeated overuse may prove to be causative.

Arthritis Caused by Systemic Diseases

Then there's arthritis produced by the systemic diseases. Common in this group is rheumatoid arthritis. The hip is only one of the joints affected in a sufferer of this debilitating disease. The deformity on x-ray in rheumatoid arthritis is often the most severe a surgeon ever sees and is unfortunately usually accompanied by unremitting pain, that often won't respond to any regimen except surgery, and sometimes not even then.

Arthritis Caused by Autoimmune Syndromes

There are also the small numbers of arthritic hips produced by other autoimmune syndromes such as lupus, rare blood dyscrasias, and psoriasis. Again, on x-ray they may be virtually indistinguishable from osteoarthritis. Hip arthritis is also associated with long-term steroid use, alcoholism, and diabetes.

These additional medical problems bring risks that both surgeon and patient must take into account.

No matter where you fit into this spectrum of arthritis, if the condition has progressed to the point that the symptoms dominate your life, it is time for surgery.

Chapter Two Highlights

- Is it your hips or something else?
- Osteoarthritis and its bearing on the subject.
- Other conditions leading to arthritis.
- Pain threshold and your decision to have surgery.

Your Space

_____

_____

_____

_____

_____

_____

_____

_____

_____

_____

The Decision to Have Surgery

Once you know you have severe hip arthritis, you may find yourself wondering if there are options other than surgery, or at least if there is something you can do to delay surgery. There are legitimate deferment and temporizing ploys, but evasion is a whole different ball game. So let's consider the options.

Hip Arthroscopy

Hip arthroscopy is one of the legitimate delay or deferment ploys. It allows you and your surgeon to get more information about your hip problem, while at the same time performing a localized treatment that may give you a safe degree of pain relief. In a nutshell, hip arthroscopy is a pain-free local "look-see."

Your doctor inspects your hip with a small bore "scope" that is inserted through an incision of about 1 centimeter long (less than 1/2 inch). A mini-camera is attached to the scope to provide the surgeon with a clear 3-D look at your hip joint.

Through a second 1-centimeter incision, an instrument about the size of a number-two pencil is also introduced into the hip. The two instruments permit the surgeon to simultaneously see and work on the joint. It may mean removing loose bodies, such as loose cartilage or fragments of bone that have detached from the joint surfaces, as well as shaving down some of the surface irregularities that arthritis has produced within the joint, and—above all—washing out the arthritic debris.

You'll get either local anesthetic or an epidural producing complete numbness. Should you feel pain you may become a moving target seriously interfering with the work your surgeon is trying to get done. Obviously it's vital to his vision and preciseness that you stay still.

Arthroscopy has several pluses in its favor, as it gives the surgeon a real and direct view of the affected hip. Hence, what to do, and when to do it, becomes an informed decision between patient and surgeon. What the surgeon sees in the arthroscope will affect his or her choice of prosthesis and even which procedure she recommends.

The cleanout in an arthroscopy may bring immediate pain relief, delaying a more definitive procedure to a time of election. Pain-modifying medication can also be instilled directly into the hip joint–pretty much a win-win deal.

However, you must understand that this is a temporizing procedure that can modify the situation but rarely, if ever, correct it.

Medication and Activity Modification

Another potential option is what I call the medication and activity modification route. There are oral medications that can safely ease the pain of a troubled hip for a time, specifically non-steroidal anti-inflammatories in combination with a moderate analgesic. I've known patients with moderate arthritic pain to do reasonably well for months, if not years, on medication. The problem is that many medications that are good for joints wreak havoc on your stomach.

How helpful is activity modification? Well, in the hundreds of patients I've been privileged to treat over the years, I've heard everything from "Yes, it helped a bit," to, "No difference at all, Doc." This last response was often accompanied by a distinctly disappointed and skeptical look. What I've never heard is, "The pain is all gone now."

If you're trapped in a pattern of repeated or increasing doses of pain meds, such as Tylenol with or without codeine, or if you're even thinking about living on a Percocet equivalent, it's time to schedule your hip procedure.

Surgery Evasion

If you decide to become essentially chair bound, limiting activities more and more to what you can accomplish with an impaired hip, it's your choice to live this way, tough love be damned. But it's really a vicious circle—the more you don't do, the more you can't do, as your muscles slowly weaken and your joint becomes more stiff and painful. Unfortunately, I know this firsthand.

Also, beware of "snake oil" medications that promise you total relief—especially those you may find online. Note the plugs for various mega-vitamin/mineral supplements and other preparations that may be advertised as "miraculous," "ancient," or "Oriental." Though they sound tempting to try, they are often unverifiable, expensive, and useless, and may even contain harmful ingredients.

Speaking of the dangers of evasion, that brings me to the ever-hot topic of steroids.

Cortisone and Other Steroids

Entire books have been written on steroids. They are mainstream treatment for rheumatoid or other autoimmune-disease patients. For the rest of us, steroids can work miraculously in terms of pain relief, putting many conventional pain relievers to shame. *But*—the stories you hear about pro athletes are all true. Consider the use of Butisoldin, a steroid that is used in racehorses (also occasionally in human beings). The horse will run until a leg breaks, because its pain is deadened. We don't permit humans to do this, but the repeated or chronic use of steroids will still result in total joint destruction in the long run. We are all too aware that long-term or repeated use of these drugs results in side effects such as:

- Fragility of bone—a minor fall can result in a major fracture.
- Susceptibility to serious infections—steroids *seriously* interfere with your immune system.
- Weight gain.
- Possible onset of diabetes.
- A rounding of the face, referred to as moon facing, and increased hair growth in unwanted locations (charming?!).

I don't think I need to go on. Just don't even think of long-term use of even small doses of a steroid as courting anything but disaster.

To be fair, your knee or hip may benefit from one or even two injections of steroid, directly into the joint. But this is altogether different from oral use in that it stays strictly local, avoiding the systemic effects listed above. However, repeated injections can produce the racehorse effect, so be very, very cautious.

Always remember that pain, whether in general, in an extremity, or in a joint, is your body's warning to you that something is amiss and must be taken seriously.

Glucosamine/Chondroitin Sulfate

There are still many advertisements in both general and medical journals about the effectiveness of glucosamine and chondroitin sulfate, taken orally or injected into an affected joint. Without discussing whether or not insurance will pay for their cost, I've yet to see an article or patient in whom they really do the job. Temporary pain relief, perhaps. Permanent pain relief, no. I've never seen any significant proof that they heal, grow, or even re-grow real cartilage to give back the normal smooth-gliding joint surface.

Other Forms of Avoidance

Worth mentioning here are "delay ploys" involving specific exercise modalities. These are dealt with in Chapter Six as part of a well-advised pre-surgical regimen. Suffice it to say that I think of them as part of permitting legitimate surgical delay.

One of the smartest things a patient can do on his own behalf is to get his body, no matter how compromised by physical problems, in the best shape possible for a surgical procedure. It makes post-operative rehabilitation and recovery that much easier.

The Benefits of Total Hip Replacement or Resurf, in a Nutshell

These may be totally clear to you if you've ever known someone who had a successful THR or Resurf. In summary, it's the difference between being handicapped, and possibly even wheelchair bound, or being part of the upright, two-legged, and walking population of this world.

Did I mention the probability of being pain-free?

- No more depending on anti-inflammatory pills in the attempt to lessen pain with Voltarin, Relafen, Motrin, Advil—or name your favorite brand—followed by antacids for the irritation of your gastrointestinal system.
- No more nights that you can't find sleep because of pain, and no more worry about moving the wrong way in bed. And have you had to use sleeping pills regularly on top everything else?

- Think of being able to join your "active" friends in most of their activities. Day-trips, extended travel, evenings out on the town, even dancing may return to your program. No more apologies to your significant other about your physical or sexual limitations.

Is Surgery the Only Real Solution?

Surgeons believe that for anatomical problems such as fractures, arthritis, et al., the solution must be anatomical, that is to say surgical. Surgery is the only thing capable of modifying anatomy.

Patients, however, may suspect that surgery is not really needed, or that the surgeon is trying to boost his or her revenue by filling the coffers with new surgeries. The bottom line is that if you need surgery, you need surgery, but this is why I also always advise second opinions.

Keep in mind that surgeons must face the results of their own surgery, be aware of reports in the medical journals, and the criteria and criticism of their colleagues. So it's not a matter of income, although it may be a matter of pride of skill.

Perspectives in Doctor-Patient Conversations

Surgeon: "A total hip replacement is major surgery and carries risks."

Patient: "How major is the risk? Is it worth my life?"

Reality: To put it in scale, the risk is less than it would be with heart bypass surgery but considerably more than a D&C (dilation and curettage), or prostate or oral surgery.

Many GPs/Internists: "I would advise that you wait until you are older to have a hip replacement, maybe 70 or 75."

Patient: "You think I should wait that long? Your hip may feel fine, doctor, but mine hurts like hell."

Reality: You must be the judge of how seriously your hip pain is affecting the quality of your life. And the advent of the Hip Resurfacing procedure is intended for a younger, active patient.

Further Reality: Initially surgeons were promising only 10 years before a THR might need to be revised. Today, THR durations of 15 to 20 years are not a bit unusual.

End of Debate

I can't think of an orthopedist who isn't willing to have a patient try physical therapy, medication, and activity modification before offering to schedule surgery. As do most of my colleagues, I have always told my patients, "You will tell me when it's time to do your THR or Resurf."

I'm sure there have been times in your life when you've said "Enough! No more!" The decision to have a THR or Resurf may well be one of them. Do I sound like I'm a THR believer? You bet I am—both as a surgeon and as a recipient! But risks do exist, and I'll talk about them in Chapter Five.

Chapter Three Highlights

Legitimate Non-surgical Options
- Medication and exercise.
- Hip arthroscopy.

Timing of Surgery
- THRs and Resurfs are elective surgeries, so it's up to you.
- Consider your pain and disability level.

Evasion of Surgery (Not recommended)

- If you put off surgery, your knees, back, and hip may pay for it.
- Muscle mass may weaken or lessen.

Your Space

_____

_____

_____

_____

_____

_____

_____

_____

_____

_____

_____

_____

Total Hip Replacement and Resurfacing– Step by Step

I t's important to have an understanding of what is actually done during your THR or Resurf surgery, and this chapter covers the basics of both procedures. If you want a blow-by-blow account of either surgery, there are brilliantly produced videos available in orthopedic offices and online as well. These videos show the surgical procedure graphically from start to finish. If you appreciate the inner workings of the human body, these videos may be for you.

Total Hip Replacement

The following are the basic steps in a THR:

Step 1: Your surgeon will make an incision, approximately 6 to 8 inches long, starting at your upper thigh and running up onto the buttock. Surgeons call this a "J" incision. (It actually looks like an inverted letter "J.")

Step 2: By careful dissection, the incision is carried down through layers of muscle and the hip capsule to gain exposure to the hip joint.

Step 3: The surgeon then removes the old hip, both ball and socket, and creates a cleaned-up, reamed-out freshened base of bone, ready for the prosthesis.

Step 4: Both cup and femoral head are usually press-fit. Boney in-growth into the stem of the femoral component is thus encouraged. There may be special circumstances that induce the surgeon to use cement to secure the femoral stem, but this is usually reserved for revisions. Your surgeon will discuss its use, should it be needed.

Step 5: I should mention the "spacesuits" worn by the surgical team, and the laminar airflow system. Their use is very important, and you should actually confirm with your surgeon in advance that they will use both of these items. The suits and laminar airflow system are used in most O.R.s to minimize the patient's exposure to possible infection.

Step 6: Antibiotics (medical protection against infection) are started intravenously as soon as you're on the table and are continued post-op for a minimum of three to five days.

Step 7: A Foley catheter will be inserted into your bladder to measure urine output, and it may be left in place for two or three days post-op. Both inflow/outflow measurements are extremely important in these first few days. You will be losing body fluids and need to have them carefully measured and replaced. The Foley makes this possible. Note that for a few days after surgery you will also have a drain placed in the hip to permit the escape and measurement of blood and fluid that would otherwise collect deep in the wound.

Step 8: You may or may not need your pre-donated blood. Your medical team will often use a blood saver, a device that collects, filters, and gives back much of the blood you lose during the time you are on the operating table.

Step 9: A trial prosthesis is inserted to check the sizing of the prosthesis and to test its stability. If stable through a range of motion, the final device is placed.

Step 10: The new prosthesis is put once more through a range-of-motion test to re-test its stability. Then the hip incision is closed from bone to skin.

Step 11: After the wound is dressed, you'll be transferred back onto a gurney and taken to the recovery room.

Step 12: Many surgeons start a sequential compression device (SCD), which is a mechanical calf squeezer, designed to discourage blood clots, right on the table. I think it's a must, especially during this immediate post-op period when you are least conscious and least active.

Step 13: On the operating table, before you're transferred to a gurney, an abduction brace will be placed between your legs to prevent dislocation of your new hip.

About the surgical incision: THR scars are not petite. They will heal side to side, not end to end, and will really flatten and fade with time. In my view, a THR or Resurf scar is a badge of courage and sense.

Hip Resurfacing

I would describe the hip resurfacing procedure as an alternative to traditional hip replacement in which the femoral head and acetabulum (hip socket) are resurfaced rather than replaced. As you know, total hip replacement requires the removal of the femoral head and the insertion of a stem down the shaft of the femur. Hip resurfacing, on the other hand, preserves the femoral head and the femoral neck, but, as its name says, it resurfaces the existing ball and socket.

During the hip resurfacing procedure, Steps 1 through 7 are virtually the same as in the THR. The last portion of a resurfacing is technically quite demanding and shows little tolerance for variation or modification from the ideal. It makes resurfing more difficult and surgeons' learning curve steeper. As the procedures are similar, especially Steps 1 through 7, the resurfacing difference begins with Step 8.

Step 8: After the surgeon dislocates the hip, the head of the hip is now preserved and re-contoured to normal congruence and measured. During the procedure the surgeon only removes a few centimeters of bone around the femoral head, shaping it tightly inside the hip-resurfacing implant.

Step 9: The acetabulum (cup portion of the hip) is reamed out in preparation for the metal cup that forms the socket portion of the ball-and-socket joint.

Step 10: The resurfacing component slides over the top of the femoral head and the acetabular component is pressed into place much like a total hip replacement would be. The trial prosthetic parts are then tried through a range of motions.

Step 11: If these trial components are congruent and stable, the surgeon then replaces them with the final prosthetic parts and cements the femoral head surfacing in place. A few surgeons will cement the cup as well as the head.

Step 12: The wound is closed using the same techniques as for a THR.

The average duration of a hip replacement or resurfacing surgery is one to two hours. Complications may add another half hour, and re-dos average 1½ to 3 hours from start to finish. However, you will not remember any of this time, which is as it should be. There's a certain mercy in unawareness.

A Word About the "Mini-Hip Procedure"

Sometimes new twists are given to old procedures. The advent of endoscopic or arthroscopic surgery spawned some tagalongs, and one of them is the so-called "mini-hip."

At its heart are the keyhole incisions into the hip region, which really shouldn't be attempted by any but the most experienced surgeons. It's held up to the surgically anxious as a mini-hip procedure but, believe me, despite sounding appealing as a "mini," it's fair to say that it's "maxi"-risky. The procedure is just as much "major" surgery as an actual hip resurfacing or replacement. The incisions are not

INSIDER TIP

About Bone Density

Whether you're contemplating a THR or a Resurf, a bone density evaluation lies somewhere between a plus and a must. You can have a simple, painless bone density test or, better yet, the whole enchilada—a FRAX.

The FRAX, which I would strongly recommend, is a fracture risk assessment tool recently introduced by the World Health Organization. It includes bone density as one of its parameters, but also uses family history, pertinent medical history, and any related calcium matters in its calculations.

Resurfs, particularly in pre-menopausal women, as noted, have a significant failure rate due to bone fragility and subsequent fracture and/or failure.

Whether you're to have a Resurf or THR, if your surgeon hasn't ordered bone density tests, he should be reminded. It certainly affects the decision whether to have a resurf, and may affect THR prostheses choice, or even the surgery itself.

A Comparison of Total Hip Replacement and Hip Resurfacing

	Total Hip Replacement	Resurfacing
Age	Usually 65 years and up	30s (if need be) to 55
Duration	15+ years; documentation available in medical literature	The jury is out; device has not been used long enough for reliable statistics
Range of Motion	Adduction and Flexion limited	No limitation
Full Weight Bearing	6 weeks	1-2 weeks
Full Athletics	Limited	Possible but not always smart
Women; Pre-Menopausal, Obesity, Rheumatoid Dysplastic Hips, Vascular Necrosis, Low Bone-Density Score	Okay	Not advisable

really keyhole sized, though they are much smaller than the standard surgical approach to the hip.

About incisions: It's not smart to insist on what is called a keyhole or mini-type incision. Yes, for the moment you will have less of a scar. However, small incisions limit a surgeon's ability to see the joint, capsule, and surrounding muscle that he is working on, which is *not* in the least desirable. In fact, using tiny incisions actually increases the possibility that a nerve or blood vessel may be inadvertently harmed. For the surgeon to have enough exposure to freely see, touch, and thus evaluate the anatomical home of your new hip is your insurance that he avoid technical mistakes which may compromise the surgical result.

Remember too, that even the largest scars can be revised by a plastic surgeon later—even before bikini season.

In essence, the ideal patient for a hip Resurf is a 55-year-old male with slight to moderate changes on x-ray, who needs to get back to work or athletics as soon as possible, and who understands that in time he may need a THR.

Recent reports in the literature indicate that women, especially those beginning to show signs of osteoporosis (thinning of bone that accompanies menopause) are poor or actually "no-go" candidates for Resurfs. There is a noticeable incidence of femoral neck fractures in these women. A THR, because of the stemmed femoral component, avoids this problem; the Resurf does not.

I do not mean to suggest that *no* women should have this procedure. But, I would definitely advise that women in their 40s have a bone density test prior to a Resurf. And I think careful consideration of family history with respect to osteoporosis is also critical. I further suggest you be a little suspicious of the fabulous stories about people who have undergone a Resurf and thereafter returned to professional athletics without later problems or limitations.

Chapter Four Highlights

- A comparison of Total Hip Replacement and Hip Resurfacing procedures.
- Which is for you—THR or Resurf?
- Beware of the misnamed "mini-hip" replacement—it may be "maxi" risky.

Your Space

_____

_____

_____

_____

_____

Complications– Theoretical and Actual

If I sound like I'm a THR and Resurfacing believer, it's because I am—both as a surgeon and a recipient. But, complications exist and you should know the theoretical and actual risks of hip surgery.

When you sit down to talk with your orthopedic surgeon about your impending hip surgery, he will discuss possible risks of the procedure. This chapter discusses what you can do to "be part of the solution" if you find yourself with one of the actual complications described here.

Can You Lose Your Life While on the Operating Table Under Anesthesia?

I find patients ask this question more frequently than any other. Surgeons sometimes treat this question as if you were a fool to raise it—which is poor perception on their part if they do so. It's neither a stupid or pointless question, and it deserves an answer. Does death from anesthesia actually occur? Yes, but fortunately it is rare as the proverbial hen's teeth and, when it does happen, it is almost invariably under general anesthesia, not under "spinals," which are preferred for THRs and Resurfs.

My research of the last eight years on THRs done in this country failed to reveal one reported incident of death under anesthesia in a normal THR candidate. I think a significant reason for this absence is the newer anesthesia techniques combined with the newer orthopedic surgical methods.

On a related note, allergy to anesthesia is a very rare risk. Modern anesthesiologists are very aware of this possibility, and, should it arise, can immediately treat it with anything from an antihistamine to epinephrine in your IV. A good anesthesiologist is constantly alert for the faintest, first sign that you're in trouble on the surgical table.

You can help avoid this risk if you remember the details of any allergy you may have and repeat them to *everyone* who will listen—doctors, nurses, technicians, anyone—but especially your anesthesiologist.

Now, what about the surgery itself? What are the most common, serious risks?

Surgical Complications

When orthopedic surgeons talk among themselves about the overall complications of THR, what they really mean is the *risk* of complications. With THRs we're talking about an occurrence of less than 2 to 3 percent. With Resurfs it's a little higher, at 3.5 to 4 percent.

However, you may get the impression that complications and risks are more frequent and disastrous than the above percentages suggest. It must be remembered that complications make for far more interesting cocktail conversations, and tabloid articles, than the far less colorful but much more satisfactory success stories. Why does a bloody serial killing get more coverage than an international peace accord?

But fair is fair, there are complications.

Accumulated Thrombus

An accumulated thrombus is a blood clot formation leading to embolism. This is the one surgeons worry about most, and it's the one that they take all kinds of precautions against, especially pulmonary.

Clot and Thrombosis Prevention

INSIDER TIP

Your surgeon and internist will choose the most effective medicine to prevent thrombosis based on their clinical experience, plus a review of medical journals and current research. Chances are they won't explain the exact chemical reactions and technical details of their choice.

But there are mechanical helpers that you should know and care about.

The sequential calf device (SCD) is a premier anti-thrombotic device. It is, in essence, a cuff applied to your operated leg from thigh to ankle. It is set up to compress the veins in your legs, gently and on a regulated cycle.

Continuous passive motion (CPM) is used to start early gentle and range-controlled hip movement. As the name implies, it is used primarily to start early hip motion, but it helps a fair bit with anti-clot formation.

Another simple anti-clot device is the elastic stocking. This fits from thigh to toe, is put on in the morning, and is removed at night. Most of my summertime patients weren't a bit patient with it. As an elective (after the SCD and CPM machines are no longer in use), it may be very helpful.

Pulmonary Embolism

During the surgery, when the bones of the hip are handled, and the prosthesis inserted, small blood clots and fat droplets are created (this can't be avoided). These clots and droplets may travel from the site of their formation into the smaller, and then greater, veins of the body, especially in the lower legs, and form thrombi. There, they can clump together into larger clots that in turn may travel on (this is what is meant by embolism). Small thrombi formed in the course of surgery are so prevalent that they have never been accurately measured. Suffice it to say that it almost always happens. The question is really: Once formed, what then?

Veins are the blood vessels that return blood to lungs, where it is oxygenated, and then to the heart for re-circulation. The important issue is how large the clots are, and where they end up if they break off. Bear in mind that veins may ease the passage of thrombi as they become larger nearing the heart and lungs.

If the clots remain small and lodged in the veins of the legs, they will in all likelihood cause no real problems—end of story! But if they accumulate and move to the larger vessels, they can arrive at the lungs and then the heart. And this last phenomenon (pulmonary embolism) is life-threatening. The trick is to prevent it from happening, and generally this can be done with anti-coagulant medication, plus calf squeezing.

There is a nationwide maximum incidence of pulmonary embolism of 2 to 3 percent in orthopedic literature. Actually, since orthopedists are exceedingly aware of events leading to embolism, each and every one has an anticoagulant program that he administers during surgery, and for a significant period afterward.

Make sure your surgeon is informed if you've ever had any problems with your veins (phlebitis, varicosities, and any other conditions relating to veins and circulation), especially if you're taking a blood thinner for any reason whatsoever. Your pre- and post-operative regimen must be adjusted accordingly.

A previous history of circulation or heart problems increases your surgical risk significantly, so they must be thoroughly treated and discussed in detail with your internist, surgeon, and anesthesiologist prior to surgery. Discuss these risks with your internist, and talk to your surgeon about his plans to protect against them during and after the surgery.

In the end, severe venous circulatory or cardiac problems may make you double think a THR despite your pain and disability. Think about it coolly, but seriously, balancing pros and cons, the risks, and benefits to you as an individual, before you decide whether to have the surgery.

Failure of Procedure—Can My Hip End Up Worse?

Medical literature (the reported results of THR) indicates that if you're the usual THR candidate, you can anticipate a result of anywhere from good to very, very good. So with reported "good" results of more than 97 percent, the chance of a poor result is slim.

Now, if you're thinking you'll receive a *perfect* joint, perhaps that's a touch too optimistic.

Is it possible that you'll continue to feel an occasional twinge after a THR? You bet it is. Could you have some residual morning stiffness? Again, yes. Might there be limitations on range of motion at the hip joint? Yes. *But*, complete failure is not a reasonable possibility. The assumption here, of course, is that you're not in the category of systemically challenged (e.g., have a neurological condition, lupus, or rheumatoid arthritis, etc.). If you are, the odds may shift.

Although the nationwide results from THR are overwhelmingly positive, you may not be a shoe-in for the Boston or New York Marathon, or for attempting an assault on a Himalayan peak. You should, however, expect to regain the ability to carry out reasonable activities of daily living, including most sports.

Infection

Search of the medical literature indicates a 1 to 2 percent post-operative infection rate. That refers to actual joint infections that may lead to the need to remove the implanted prosthesis. Many of these infections are related to high-risk patient groups, such as those with diabetes or patients who've been on steroids long-term, or whose immune systems are compromised.

- Ask your chosen surgeon about his or her specific infection rate.
- Ask your chosen surgeon what precautions will be taken against infection
- Prophylactic antibiotic administration is a basic precaution.

Excessive Blood Loss

THR is a major procedure, and in the course of surgery there is almost unavoidably a considerable amount of blood loss. Your surgeon will tell you that you can and should pre-donate your own blood two weeks before surgery. Then, if and when needed, it's available to give back to you on the operating table.

Actually, most surgeons also use a blood-saver system, which recaptures some of the blood you lose during surgery, and, under sterile conditions, restores a portion of it back to you right then and there. Careful surgical technique in performing the procedure is key, minimizing the need for blood administration.

Transfusion Problems

There are fewer transfusion problems now than there were in the 1980s when AIDS was a significant consideration. Careful screening and testing by blood banks has almost eliminated this hazard. Still, the possibility of hepatitis C remains, so your best course of action is to pre-plan and pre-donate.

Post-Operative Pneumonia

This used to be a real consideration for all major surgical

procedures—the result of post-operative inactivity combined with being kept in bed for extended periods after surgery. Today, surgeons insist that you get up and out of bed the day after surgery and *move!*

There is also a very simple hand-held gizmo called a blow bag (the official "hospitalese" for this is an incentive spirometer), which you blow into after taking a deep breath—classier than using a brown paper bag, but it serves the same purpose of keeping your lungs clear. It helps measurably against post-op pulmonary problems. By taking a deep breath and blowing out as hard as you can, you expand your lungs, moving residual accumulations of air and fluid.

Some of this aggressive post-op "up-and-out-of-bed" routine is due to the fact that third-party payers have reduced the post-op in-hospital days they will cover for a given procedure. There are times that insurers and healthcare providers are in synch to the benefit of the patient. This is one of them.

Needless to say, antibiotic coverage also has a significant role in preventing pulmonary infections.

Sciatic Nerve Palsy

More of a nuisance than a hazard is sciatic nerve palsy. Occasionally patients find they have numbness and some weakness in the operated leg. During the procedure, sometimes the large nerve that supplies sensation and motor power down the leg may get bruised or stretched. This condition is short-lived and doesn't result in permanent nerve palsy.

Sciatic nerve palsy may result in a foot or toe drop due to operative pressure or stretch. Usually this condition resolves within a matter of weeks. If permanent (which is really rare), an ankle brace in the shoe compensates for the foot drop. Leg length equality is one of the areas an experienced orthopedist focuses on intently during both pre-op planning and measurement and intra-operative execution. Very minor inequality in leg lengths—even if not needing correction—may lead to *tem-*

porary peroneal nerve weakness. Leg-length inequality of 1/2 inch or less may have been the tradeoff for prosthetic stability. More than 1/2 inch may require a small shoe lift.

Heterotopic or Ectopic Calcification

This condition is rarely seen today, possibly due to the careful and aggressive washout during surgery that's now possible with the Waterpik. This device provides thorough, forceful lavage to the joint and surrounding tissue, removing boney debris created during prosthetic implantation to a minimum. It is a tool used assiduously by virtually all hip surgeons.

Ectopic calcification, which can be detected on x-rays, is often asymptomatic, needing nothing more than observation. Typically the calcification forms in the abductor muscle, or the lateral aspect of the hip joint. If it begins to create pressure tenderness, or—in instances so rare as to be reportable—it interferes with hip abduction, it is surgically removed and/or treated with irradiation or steroids.

Dislocation

Dislocations do happen, and THR surgeons have a difficult time dealing with some of the implications. In the so-called "neurologic" group of patients (those who have Parkinson's disease, cerebral palsy, epilepsy, and others), dislocation is a common and known risk that both patient and surgeon accept in the attempt to allay severe hip pain.

If a patient falls in the immediate post-op period or disobeys or forgets instructions not to over-bend or turn the hip inward, a dislocation may result. There is usually a clear cause-and-effect sequence when such a dislocation occurs.

In the absence of a precipitating event (post-operative fall, accident, or trauma), or some problem known and discussed pre-operatively, the surgeon is faced with the implication of sub-optimal technique. I leave you to imagine it is not a favorite review topic with orthopedists. On the other hand, Resurfs have a negligible incidence of dislocation due to any cause.

In any case, such a dislocation means the patient will be put under a light anesthesia while the surgeon manipulates the hip back into place. Afterwards, the patient will spend a period of time in an abduction brace to keep the hip from turning inward.

A far more grievous problem is recurrent dislocation. If dislocation repeats within the year, or several times within the next few years, the hip must be re-operated to stabilize it against continuing episodes.

You are mostly in control of most common cause of dislocations. You're told point blank that for the first 6 to 12 weeks you must avoid excessive hip flexion and adduction at all costs, as these are the immediate cause of dislocations.

Technical Complications

The New Metal-on-Metal Dilemma

There is no definitive answer as to which type of hip implant is the "best." The reason for this is that in order to evaluate the long-term success of implants, studies need to continue for many years and include many patients to truly understand their impact—both positive and negative.

Until the last few years, the hip prosthesis consisted of a metal head fit into a "polyethylene" cup. The life of the prosthesis was put at 10 or 15 years of use before it would *possibly* need to be replaced.

Then, in seeking increased stability and device longevity, and also to help patients avoid a second surgical procedure, biomechanical researchers suggested that a larger metal head fitted into a metal cup would accomplish these ends. Thus many manufacturers both here and abroad produced a metal-on-metal device, giving surgeons this choice. The metal-on-metal (MonM) addressed the problem of dislocation (one of the most common replacement complications). The metallic femoral head was thought to glide smoothly on the metallic acetabular surface. This new implant would allow the patient to have a THR at a younger age, while still avoiding the possibility of a late-life replacement due to the device's extended longevity. It seemed logical. It seemed a *great* solution.

However, recent experience with the metal-on-metal prosthesis has produced significant reports of metal debris with use. This debris then must be handled by the body—it may be absorbed into the blood stream, or it may accumulate in or around the hip joint, neither of which is a desirable phenomenon. And quoting recent studies of the problem, "friction" produced between head and cup has led to inflammatory reactions, and to such phenomena as death of tissue in the hip joint, loss of surrounding bone, and pain.

Metal-on-metal prostheses are also subject to "edge loading," which can occur when the metal prosthetic head butts up against the top edge of the metal cup, producing even more microscopic metal debris over time. This is exacerbated when the patient rises from a chair or climbs stairs. I think you can see without aid what distance jogging or running might produce.

It is not clear what percentage of metal-on-metal patients may be affected or how long it may take for problems to appear. What seems sure is that these patients may need a replacement sooner than expected. Ironically, this is just the problem metal-on-metal devices were meant to solve.

From the point of view of risk, in light of the medical research of the last few years and recent implant recalls, metal-on-metal THRs or resurfs constitute a major, avoidable risk! If there's one technical subject to discuss with your surgeon prior to surgery, this is it. I had used, and still advise, a metal femoral part of a polyethylene acetabulum for the usual procedure. Until something really better comes along, this is the way to go.

Remember, Only God Makes the Perfect Hip

Orthopedic surgeons are always looking for improved methods and materials for hip replacement and/or resurfacing. But there is a basic problem in striving for these. In order to know how good a prosthesis really is, one has to observe and analyze it for between 8 and 10 years. But, if the newer implant seems to offer marked advantages early on, and there are no obvious or immediate problems, both patients and surgeons want to use it immediately.

Hip replacement implants have been modified over the years in order to provide the best possible function—with long-lasting results. There are many hip implant designs available to surgeons. There is no absolute consensus on what is the best prosthetic design.

In trying for better implants, some glitches have occurred with several implants.

- In the titanium femoral and acetabular implant, the metal didn't hold up well against weight-bearing stress.
- A ceramic-on-ceramic implant led to easier dislocations.
- The metal-on-metal devices have produced metal debris that is absorbed into the body, and the friction between the head and cup can produce inflammatory reactions.

Your Own Contribution to Surgical Risk

Contribution to surgical risk on your behalf can be summed up in a word or two: a less-than-complete medical history. If your surgeon and your anesthesiologist are unaware of something that puts you at risk, they can only play catch-up if anything unfavorable occurs. This is not the position they or *you* want to be in.

Don't worry that your surgeon may refuse to do the THR if he knows you're a tricky patient. If he's experienced, he will know how to handle your case. But if he and the anesthesiologist are not completely informed of your condition, you could be subjected to unacceptable risk!

Please don't rely wholly on your internist to convey your medical history. He or she probably will, but always err on the side of caution, and never feel embarrassed if you think you may be repeating information.

If you fail to heed post-op instructions by turning your hip inward or over flexing, you could cause the most common THR problem—dislocation.

If you neglect anticoagulation meds post-op, you may end up with clotting problems, which can be truly serious. It's really upsetting when unfortunate outcomes could have been avoided, both for the patient and the surgeon, so be sure to communicate.

Now, even as you want your surgeon to listen to you, when she explains or describes something, don't simply wait for your turn to talk; *really listen to what she has to say*, both before and after your surgery. Take in the answers to your questions. This is an essential part of any two-way conversation and doubly important when the subject concerns your surgery.

One of my fourth-year medical students once said to me in wonder, "Man, like, patients are like people!" I remind you as gently as possible, "like, surgeons are like people, too," and under no circumstances are they to be confused with unquestionable gods.

Post-Op Patient Contribution to Complications

This is the time that you become a major player on your own behalf. It is the time that you become part of the solution, not the problem. You must become the real partner in the project of your own welfare. So far, by and large, your surgeon has carried the burden and provided the solution to your hip problem. Now it's your turn.

In order to complete your surgery safely and make the transition back to normalcy, you are *must* to do two things: ***observe and report*** *any of the following:*

Thrombi or Pulmonic Emboli

For the first 6 to 12 weeks after hip surgery, thrombi and pulmonic emboli are and should be a subject of your serious and consistent attention. Remember that deep vein thrombosis or clot formation can lead to pulmonary emboli, which *are life-threatening.*

It's true that one or both of these things may occur no matter what you and your surgeon do. But the likelihood that you will suffer such an occurrence is markedly lessened by the following:

- Starting an immediate post-op anti-coagulating routine, with an IV anti-coagulating agent and oral medication (e.g., Warfarin, Coumadin or, my preferred, aspirin) or one of the newer anti-coagulatory medications (see your internist).
- Using a PCA calf-squeezing machine.
- Doing frequent sets of calf-muscle exercise.

Perhaps the most important deterrent to pulmonary emboli is *your early detection of the symptoms,* such as:

- Calf pain, swelling, even redness—this needs immediate attention.
- Shortness of breath, dry cough, or chest pain—these are emergencies.

In my own practice I hoped for the following when my post-op patients went home:

- The use of an adult dose (325mg) aspirin twice a day. Not for those with ulcer problems—your internist will substitute.
- Rental and use at night of a PCA machine for the first month (automated calf-massaging device).
- Elevation of leg whenever possible and frequent calf exercises.

Infection

Infections are reported as long as 12-plus weeks after surgery. The source or cause is not always clear. What is clear is that the sooner they are identified and treated, the better.

In the hospital you were on antibiotics given initially by IV, then orally. In general this would be the first five days after surgery. If, however, you develop a superficial wound infection, it will be treated in the hospital with topical antibiotics or a superficial incision and drainage procedure, accompanied by repeated cultures of the site.

In the rare instance that you might develop a deep wound infection during this time, you would be taken to the O.R. and your hip joint lavaged through an arthroscope. Antibiotics would be instilled directly into the surgical site (with suitable cultures taken to assure that the infection was susceptible to the antibiotic chosen).

If signs and symptoms of infection disappear and cultures and blood studies come back clean, that's it. If, on the other hand, repeated cultures are still positive, and other studies are not satisfactory, the surgeon will determine the continuing treatment. The jury is out on what further treatment is optimal. It may mean an immediate prosthetic replacement or a delayed one.

Now, after you go home: *Any ooze from your incision area— even if clear—must be treated as an infection.* Your surgeon must see it promptly. It is your further job to insist to whomever answers the office phone that you must be seen immediately.

This is no time to win friends and influence people! You are to be seen—not in a week or the earliest opening—*now!*

Post-Op Pain

Remember that your body has undergone major surgery. Some patients do complain of moderate pain for the first week or two post op. Usually it is the diminishing kind—sometimes at night, sometimes at the end of the day, or even at the beginning of the day.

But at 12 weeks there should normally be no pain. If there remains significant or even increasing pain (and by this time a patient knows what that is), your surgeon will take an x-ray to check for the following possibilities:

- Loosening of the prosthesis.
- Infection (unheralded by ooze or fever). See section on post-op infection.
- Referred pain (needing intense physical therapy).
- Possible allergy to metal.
- Early debris formation.

The last two possibilities (allergy to metal and early debris formation) have no standard treatment as of this writing.

Lastly, remember to follow daily activity safety rules and precautions you have learned.

Chapter Five Highlights

- The least important is anesthesia.
- The most important is pulmonary embolism (traveling post-op blood clots).
- The new metal-on-metal dilemma.

Your Space

_____

_____

_____

_____

_____

_____

_____

_____

_____

_____

_____

_____

_____

_____

_____

_____

Choosing Your Medical Team and Scheduling Your Surgery

C hoosing your surgeon is one of the most difficult—and important—decisions regarding surgery of the hip, or, for that matter, any kind of surgery.

If you have an internist (medical specialist) in whom you have confidence, or with whom you have an ongoing or long-term relationship, he may want to suggest an orthopedic surgeon. His medical judgment is certainly better than that of a friend of a friend, or someone you've "heard" is "the best." The M.D. grapevine is likely a lot better than yours! Additionally, your internist and the surgeon may practice in the same hospital, which is a must if you want your own internist to follow your post-op course, which is a very good idea.

How to Find and Research Potential Surgeons

What if your internist is not able to recommend an orthopedic surgeon? Again, I'd like to emphasize that the chanciest way to choose a surgeon is to take the word of a friend, or a friend of a friend. I know, friends are there to help you when you need them, and it seems natural to turn to them, but don't go this route. You could just wind up losing a friend and being on the losing end of a less-than-great operative result. You would basically be letting someone, however well intended, with no medical expertise or knowledge, make a critical medical choice. If your friend has had a THR or Resurf, it's better information, but not necessarily a solid judgmental basis or range of experience.

My first suggestion is to look up potential choices of orthopedic surgeon through your state or county medical society, or on the Internet (using the search terms "THR" or "Hip Resurfacing").

At the very least you'll know if he's an orthopedic surgeon, a joint replacement specialist, how many years he's been in practice, where he trained, and what his hospital associations are. A word of caution, however: There are just as many sources of misinformation on the Internet as there are sources of accurate information, so use this route at your own risk and be sure to verify information you find with sources outside the Internet.

My second suggestion is to set up an appointment and interview the surgeon you think you want. (See sidebar "Questions to Ask Your Potential Surgeon.")

Another suspect or unwise way to pick a surgeon is by what hospital you think you'd like to be in. Don't pick a hospital, and then choose a doctor who is available at that hospital. This would be in the reverse order of importance. You may be housed more fashionably, and possibly get better bedside service, but that's small change compared to the outcome of your surgery.

By the way, if you're curious, ask to see a model of the hip implant your surgeon plans to use. He'll most likely have such a model on his desk. If you happen to be the nuts-and-bolts type, your surgeon will most likely have a video of the procedure available as well as a working model in the office.

Questions to Ask Your Potential Surgeon

Among the questions you can and *should* ask your surgeon are:

- How many years have you been doing the procedure?
- Where did you get your THR training?
- How many THRs did you perform last year? And the year before?
- What is your complication rate?
- What do you see as possible complications in my case? (These should obviously be consistent with those your internist has identified.)
- What hospital will you use and why? (You're looking for heavy numbers of hip surgeries done.)
- What is your upcoming schedule like? (You may not wish to wait months before having surgery.)
- What anesthesiologist and what anesthetic method will you use?
- What's covered by my insurance, and what may not be?

These are just some ideas. There may be other questions you want to ask. You may have more than one interview with your surgeon, and additional questions may pop up at this time. The point is that you should ask any questions that are meaningful to you, whether or not they may seem medically naïve or even foolish. Do not be afraid of appearing ignorant or ill-informed. You are not the doctor. It's his job to know and supply answers, not yours!

There are several implants (both for THRs and Resurfs) that are state of the art or at least have a good track record. Ask which type your surgeon intends to use. Your prosthesis should have a good clinical history of use. My own THR happened to be a Corail (invented by some very clever French doctors and brought into the United States by one of the leading orthopedic companies). Combined with the experience and technique of my surgeon, it has given me a super result.

You may ask your surgeon if you could speak to some of his previous Resurf or THR patients. By and large this would be more than fine by most surgeons, but for the sticky issue of patient confidentiality (Health Insurance Portability and Accountability Act of 1996, or HIPAA). For some surgeons, HIPPA may bar this informational route.

Be clear that you expect your internist

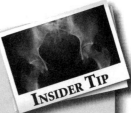

INSIDER TIP

Strike Up a Conversation with a Post-Op Patient

While you are waiting to see the surgeon, you may notice some post-op patients likewise waiting. There is nothing to prevent you from asking about their experience. Patient comments are often interesting, to the point, and helpful in understanding the whole process from the point of view of a recent recipient of a THR or Resurf. But keep in mind that the surgeon's and the patient's views of the same surgical event may vary by 180 degrees. After all, they are two different people with two different perspectives. *(My experience in this* vade mecum *is the exception: Remember, I have performed many THR surgeries and also undergone two of my own as a patient, so it is likely that my perspective as a patient and that of my surgeon were much more in sync than most!)*

and surgeon to remain in communication throughout the period of your THR. It is a sign that you have a grasp of one essential element of the procedure—communication—and this will be respected as setting the tone for the entire surgical and recovery period. They will appreciate the fact that you take a positive interest and some direction in your own case, especially if they don't already have an established relationship as medical colleagues.

Bear in mind there may be a perfectly legitimate secondary interest on the part of your surgeon, particularly if he and your internist are not well acquainted. Your surgeon *never* has a broad enough patient referral base, and is always interested in broadening it by doing a good job with a new or less-than-familiar colleague.

Don't forget to ask about how and when arrangements can be made for you to pre-donate blood. It is really somewhat up to you to form your medical team. Dr. Anesthesiologist must talk to Dr. Internist, who in turn must be in communication with Dr. Surgeon about you and your medical needs. All three must be willing and able to talk to each other and to you. This is not impossible, a luxury, or unheard of; it's important and not as hard as you think to make happen. It's just a matter of insisting that Dr. Internist talk to Dr. Anesthesiologist or Dr. Surgeon. Give the doctor 48 hours after your request for this to happen. Then ask Dr. Internist what Dr. Surgeon had to say. If this doesn't work the first time, try it a second time. If after this point it still hasn't happened, I personally would make it clear that someone isn't giving your proposed surgery the thought it deserves, walk away, and start afresh with a new team.

I can promise you that there are plenty of capable doctors willing to talk to you and each other, and who understand the importance of communicating, not only for your reassurance, but also for sound medical reasons. (This is especially important if you have a medical condition that needs any kind of special attention or consideration, e.g., diabetes, cardiac, or circulatory problems.)

I opted for, and suggest that you should also want, a surgeon with heavy experience in THRs and Resurfs. I would suggest someone who has successfully performed many of these surgeries in the past five years. No one, including surgeons, wants to repeat unsatisfactory experiences. No one, especially surgeons, like to be seen by colleagues, or even themselves, to fail at something.

In checking out the medical literature on surgeons' experience, I found that 80 percent of those performing THRs perform fewer than 15 to 20 per year. I might suggest, if you have the choice, that you find a surgeon with heavier experience than this. Since Resurfs are a newer procedure, there are even fewer surgeons with extensive experience with that procedure. Below are a few reasons *why* and *why not* to consider a prospective surgeon:

- Do not, as a general rule, choose a chairman of the department, no matter how renowned. Remember, chairpersons in the medical world are hired for their knowledge and distinction without question—but also for being good at administration! This also means they may not be as adept at performing a THR procedure as some of the members of their department who perform the operation on a more day-to-day basis.
- Personally, I would not choose a surgeon with a cold personality who appears to be bothered or annoyed by your questions, no matter what his reputation. Even if your questions are old-hat to him, they are not to you. You don't need the added stress that lack of information and an "attitude" may bring, on top of your surgery.
- It's you and only you, not your cousin Tilly, who are consenting and then undergoing major surgery—not your surgeon. You have a perfect right to know as much as possible, or certainly as much as you wish, about what is about to happen to your body.
- If you forget or don't understand an answer, don't feel embarrassed to repeat a question. If you have the spirit

Who Chooses or Suggests Your Surgeon

Source	Advantage	Disadvantage	My Rating
Family MD	Knows you and your medical problems	May not know enough about surgery and surgeons	C+
HMO	Cost covered	Only within the system or associated surgeons	C-
Friends	Frankness	No scientific basis or judgment	D
Internet (WebMD)	Accurate formal training and apts.	Data facts are one thing, skill and judgment another	B-
AAOS Listing	Experience in your locality	Still, who's for YOU?	B+
100 Best Doctors	Makes for good reading	Who pays for articles?	C
Golf/tennis pro who had procedure	Understands post-op needs	Not a surgical pro	B

and time to undergo a THR, your surgeon should have the spirit and patience to repeat answers for you. He may, at this point (fair is fair) ask you to write things down. Or he may offer you a patient information booklet. Take it and read it. If it raises further questions, your surgeon should again answer these.

- If you are a member of an HMO, you may still have a choice of surgeon. All the points I've raised in the paragraphs above still apply. If there's not a surgeon experienced in THR in your particular group, there is usually a referral list of joint replacement specialists who accept payment from your group.

- Does a surgeon have the right or responsibility to turn you down? Yes, if he considers you too grave a surgical risk or in some way on his "contradicted" list. Patients on my own list of whom I felt were contradicted for THR included those who were chronically infected, emotionally unstable (uncontrolled/uncontrollable) with serious cardiac problems or diabetes, on dialysis (urinary failure), or with severe motor or sensory neurologic disorders. On my "problematic" list were patients with severe blood dyscrasias (especially anemias), extreme obesity (200-plus pounds over normal weight), and those who were severely neurologically affected or psychologically challenged.

Keep in mind that these were my lists. Other orthopedic surgeons may feel differently.

In the end, there is no foolproof way to choose who gets to "do you." Cost may be the ultimate factor; your insurance or HMO may be another. But there's no substitute for your feeling after interviewing at least two experienced surgeons. Trust your own judgment. It's an excellent—let me correct that—probably the *best* guide, given a chance. And, the only full "A" rating I know!

Scheduling Your Surgery

Remember, although it may not feel like it, a THR is an elective procedure. That means that not only do you get to choose *whether* you will have the surgery, but also *when* it will occur. This should be worked out not to the convenience of your surgeon, but to *your* needs and convenience. Schedule it to your own calendar, giving the surgeon some leeway. It's your call. Of the choices that are in your hands, timing certainly is entirely yours. So make your scheduling decision while taking the following into consideration:

- Work absence and/or coverage. Your boss (even if you're self-employed!) will want some input.
- Pet- or house-sitting.
- Convenience or needs of significant others.
- Season—not over Christmas and New Year's, and absolutely never in July, which is when the new medical house staff comes on duty.

- Consult whomever you will be relying on to help you with your affairs for a good week or two.

Also, you don't want to find that your surgeon is on holiday or due to attend a medical conference the week after your THR is performed. He, and no one else, should follow your post-op surgical course. Of course, the same applies to your internist. And there may be other factors which play in for you, but in any case, plan out this period.

Chapter Six Highlights

- Choose a surgeon who has a successful and frequent record of hip surgeries.
- Choose a surgeon who is willing to communicate with you.
- Don't take the recommendation of your best friend.

Your Space

_____

_____

_____

_____

_____

_____

_____

_____

Pre Surgery–
A Busy Time For You

The weeks before your surgery, the preoperative (pre-op), is a time in which you can and should exert control. For those of you used to being in charge, the reasons will be evident. For those a little less accustomed to executive decisions and administrative planning, try it out.

Planning in the pre-op period gives you a grip and a sense of helping yourself that little else does. You can take charge of the event at a time when your body is not letting you control all that you'd like it to. Another plus is that planning and working on your own behalf helps calm pre-op jitters, acknowledged, unacknowledged, and even unconscious.

Second Opinions

Second opinions are mandated for most surgical procedures, including THRs, Resurfs, and hip arthroscopy. Actually, second opinions have always been a good idea for elective surgery of any kind. Surgeons almost fear the patient who in effect says, "Just do it, Doc. I trust you all the way!" and really doesn't want to hear any more whys, wherefores, caveats, or details. Get a second opinion, and—if you wish—a third. But any more than that and you're just asking for chaos and confusion; it will do nothing to clarify or amplify your decision.

Your medical insurer will require you to get a formal second opinion from an MD. If you don't get one, they may not pay for your THR.

The Issue of Weight Loss

Anything you can do to lose a few extra pounds in the months and weeks before you have surgery will help enormously. Having less weight to portage makes getting up on your feet and re-learning to walk that much easier. And in the long run, losing weight may lengthen the life of your THR.

Get help if you need it, from a dietitian, a nutritionist, or a physician. Even 10 pounds makes a difference. I, who love to eat and was living in Paris—center of the best kind of cuisine— dropped significant pounds pre-op, knowing what a difference it would make to my recovery.

As a plus, both your surgeon and anesthesiologist will be delighted, as shedding some weight will greatly reduce your operative risks. There are many anesthesiologists who will not take on a patient who is "morbidly obese," defined as twice-plus the weight for someone of a similar build.

Prehab Exercise

Exercising both "Prehab" (before surgery), and "Posthab" (after surgery) to strengthen and restore your normal hip motion and to help you gradually return to everyday activities is important for your full recovery.

There are some differences between what you *should* do and what you will *be able* to do.

Pre-operatively, the quantity of your exercise and perhaps the quality may be limited by pain. Once your surgery is performed, you will be able to do more, as your pain will be minimal to none.

Your doing prehab exercises is one of the most promising factors your surgeon can ask for; it predicts a great mindset on the part of his junior partner—*you!*

Exercising prehab has the goal of getting your muscles in the best shape you can, so that your postoperative recovery will be faster and permit you to do more sooner. The ultimate goal is to return to full activity with a few notable caveats. Think of it like the pianist who always warms up with scales and exercises that limber and prepare his fingers for work on Chopin or Liszt.

There are two main areas of exercise that I recommend pre-surgical hip patients take part in: Aqua Exercise and Non-Aquatic Core Exercise. These exercises are part of a super prep for the procedure. Granted, exercising can be tough when you're in pain and your knees and hips—not to mention your back—are stiff. You can ask your surgeon to refer you to a physical therapist who can give you a set of pre-surgical exercises that are within your scope.

The first objective of exercising pre-surgically is to keep as much range of motion as is possible in all joints, and to maintain muscle tone in general. If you have managed this as a life-long habit, I apologize for the reminder. However, if you have slowly abandoned some—if not most—exercise due to the limitations of your arthritis, I hope to encourage you to pursue exercise in a pool, or even in a chair. But keep doing as much as possible.

Your Prehab program will include strengthening your arms and shoulders, which will help you cope with crutches or a walker after surgery. It will also help maintain the strength of your leg muscles. The exercises should take about 20 minutes to complete, and if possible, you should do them twice a day.

Having said this, don't get into the "no pain, no gain" mode. Gentleness is the key. Avoid anything that produces marked pain. But you can certainly anticipate some soreness the day after a good workout.

Aqua Exercise

Exercise, as you know, comes in three general categories: aerobic, range of motion, and muscle toning. For me, both pre- and post-surgery, the nearest heated pool was heaven. I have always tried to get all of my pre-op patients to do what I call "Water Works," or water exercise. Think about it: Laps provide the perfect aerobic workout, and exercise in place provides the safest anti-gravitational environment I know for the joint-challenged. There will usually be someone associated with the pool who can teach you the specifics of range of motion and toning. Start slowly, and build reps gradually.

Other sources of information are your local arthritis foundation, state medical society, or the Internet (start with a search for aqua-aerobics).

If by any chance you have access to a heated pool, that's great. Use it. Do what you can within your range of motion. And since you are virtually weightless in the water, do a lot of running in place. Swimming laps of whatever stroke you can manage is an aerobic plus. Some gyms have saunas or steam rooms, so use them as treats after you've done your "work." Your local neighborhood pool will also be a terrific help in your post-op rehabilitation.

Non-Aquatic Core Exercise

There are legions of exercise and conditioning handbooks and manuals providing clear, complete programs. They can be used with good results.

In this section, for both convenience and specificity, I share a core series of simple lower-extremity and back exercises I always asked my patients to work on. They are calculated to strengthen what I think of as the relevant muscles of the back and legs for the THR surgery to come.

Relevant Terms

You may hear lots of semi-technical terms bantered about by therapists, doctors, or even in books devoted to exercise and physical therapy. In case you're not familiar with physical therapy jargon, let's de-mystify.

- Abduction: Moving a limb away from the center of your body.
- Adduction: Bringing a limb toward the center of your body, (in the case of hips this would mean actually crossing your legs).
- Aerobic: Any exercise that increases the heart and respiratory rates. (Often referred to as cardiovascular exercise)
- Extension: The straightening of your knee, hip, or other joint.
- Fitness Equipment: Anything from simple weighted pulley types to space-age, cyber-driven, bigger-than-a-broom-closet, mechanical whistle-and-bell machines. Fitness equipment should be used with great caution and full instruction before mounting.
- Flexion: The bending of your knee, hip, elbow, or any other joint.
- Isometric: An exercise of the joint in which the muscle is tensed without other motion; e.g. straight leg rises
- Isotonic: An exercise in which the muscle is put through a range of motion; e.g. knee flexion.
- Occupational Therapist: An occupational therapist will get you your ADL equipment and teach you how to use it. For example, she can provide you with a grabber to pick up objects from the floor.
- Physical Therapist: A physical therapist will teach you exercises and how to carry out activities of daily living (ADL), including how to use crutches, get in and out of chairs, beds, cars, etc. with safety.
- Range of Motion: Refers to the number of degrees you can

move a given joint.

- Repetition (Rep): One full specific exercise.
- Sets of Exercise: Refers to a specific number of repetitions of a given exercise. You determine how many reps a set will consist of.
- Social Worker: The social worker oversees your entire transition from hospital to home, including equipment, home nursing appointments, home physical therapy, and transportation to your home from the hospital.
- Stretching: Stretching can be isotonic or isometric, but is usually Isotonic.
- Toning: This is more or less a lay term and is the result of both of the above types of exercises, but especially isometric.

I am going to present them as exercise units. The idea is to start with one unit of each and gradually build up to about five or six units with increasing resistance (added weights).

Many of these exercises are performed in a chair. Why? There are several reasons:

- You are basically safe in a chair, and you can perform your conditioning exercises (once properly shown), securely on your own.
- For prehabs you will be able to do some really helpful muscle conditioning.
- A chair will support the parts of your body that need to be supported, so that you can concentrate on the muscles you want to exercise. (This is true in both pre- and posthab.)
- In a chair you can condition without fear of injury (especially for gung-ho posthabs; after all, it's tempting to do too much now that it doesn't hurt).
- For posthabs, the control you gain in chair exercises will help you move on to standing exercises and walking with appropriate confidence.

Quadriceps Sitting Kicks (major thigh walking muscles—front of leg)

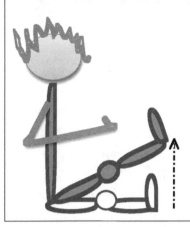

- Sit in a chair, with your back well supported.

- Extend and straighten each leg (don't bend knee).

- Lift the extended leg in a series of 10 repetitions (reps).

- Over 2 to 3 weeks, try to work up to, say, 50 reps per leg.

Quadriceps Isotonic Sitting Kicks with Weights

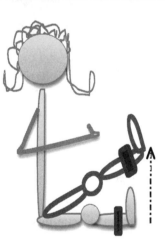

Go out to the nearest sports equipment store and buy a set of graduated Velcro ankle weights, up to but no more than 5 to 10 pounds.

- Sit in a chair; place a 1-pound ankle weight on the leg to be exercised.
- Extend and straighten each leg (as above)—start with 10 reps— gradually work up to 50.
- Next, add another 1 pound (now 2 pounds total)—start with 10 reps—gradually build up to 50 reps per leg.
- The formula works as you continue to add weight.

If you're in really great shape, go to 50 reps daily at 5 to 10 pounds of weight. There is no reason to go beyond this. If you're not accustomed to this much exercise, or don't get to more than 30 or 40 naked reps (without weight), that's fine too.

Gastrocs (major calf muscle) Isotonic Calf Press

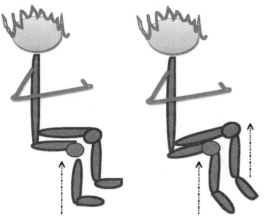

- Sit in a chair with your back well supported.
- Your legs should be in a normal sitting position.
- Go up on your toes, hold for a slow count of three, then relax.
- Start with 10 reps.
- Work up over 2 to 3 weeks to 50 reps.

Gastrocs Isotonic Calf Press with Weights

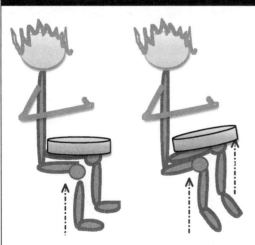

To add resistance to this exercise:

- Sit in chair; simply lean forward and put some weight on your knees.
- Do 10 reps.
- Work up gradually to 50 reps.

- Lean more of your weight on your knees, drop back to 10 reps.
- Work to 50, always adding more leaning weight.

Again, there is no special end point.

Gluteus Maximus (buttocks) Squeeze

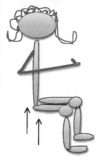

This is tricky to describe, but easy to do:

- Sit in a chair; your back should not touch the back of the chair.
- Your back should be straight up.
- Simply tighten your butt muscles (a sort of clench); if performing it correctly you will feel yourself "rise" slightly in the chair.
- Hold. Count slowly to 10 and relax.
- As in the above exercises, work up gradually to 50 reps.

Abductor Sets (big muscles on the side of your thighs)

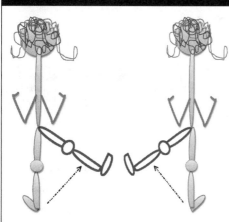

For this one, I would like you to leave your chair. Find something sturdy that can serve to support while leaving your lower body free—like the back of a sturdy chair, kitchen table, or anything that can serve as the barre used by ballet dancers.

- Stand in front of your chosen support with your upper body leaning toward it.
- Lift one leg away from your stance out to the side about 30 or 40 degrees (side leg lifts).
- Hold for a slow count of three.
- Then relax and let the leg come to neutral.
- Start with 5 to 10 reps.
- Now go to the other leg and repeat.

Gradually work up to 20 to 30 reps per side.

Abdominal Squeeze (muscular guard to your back)

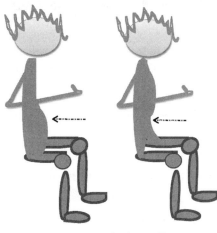

As you can see this is not, strictly speaking, a leg exercise, but a strong back helps immeasurably with walking and standing, to go along with your new hip. Core devotees take note.

- Sit in a chair with your back well supported.
- Contract your Abs by pulling your stomach right back to your spine (suck your stomach in).
- Do not hold your breath during this unit.
- Hold for a count of 10, release, and breathe.
- Start with a series of 10 reps and build to 50 reps.

Triceps ("Chair Pushups")

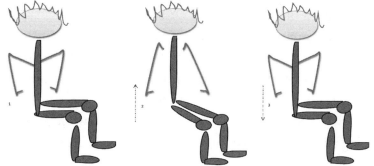

- Sit on a sturdy chair with arms.
- Grasp the arms of the chair.
- Push down on the chair arms, straightening your elbows so that you raise your buttocks off the seat.
- Lower yourself slowly back into the chair. If your arms are weak at first, use your legs to help raise your buttocks off the chair.

All of these are easy to do wherever you find yourself. They are specific for the purpose of strengthening the muscles that are either used by the hip or protective of it.

You're very wise to make these exercises a part of your pre-planning; your surgeon and physical therapist will be delighted.

The Importance of Rest

The usual understanding of rest is a cessation of activity or even awareness. It has a positive connotation, and well it should. Do we not deserve it after a task or test well done? Do we not expect it nightly as the ultimate restorative? Do we not describe something in the most positive way as being restful? Let's hear it for *rest!*

As you might guess, I'm making a point about rest as a positive element of exercise. Virtually any form and variety of rest will do.

When you start an exercise program, I would like you to try for a number of repetitions followed by a brief period of rest for several reasons:

- You will actually extend the amount of exercise you can do at a given time.
- It gives your muscles a chance to recover before being asked for more activity (I won't bother you with the chemical explanation for the phenomenon, as there has always been some disagreement about it.)
- It gives rhythm and cadence to the endeavor while providing an easy way to count sets or units of exercise.

The Matter of Private Nursing

Some major insurers cover private nursing, if your surgeon thinks it warranted. If not, and if you can afford it, it is an unqualified bonus for the first 72 hours in the hospital. Washing, dressing, transferring, general convenience, and even communication with the floor staff become much easier.

When: Call the nursing office at the hospital about two to three weeks prior to your admission. I used both day and night shifts for the first three to four days. But remember, I'd just had both sides done simultaneously and was pretty helpless and full of tubes for 72 hours.

Compensation: The nurse will ask you for payment immediately after her shift, which is usually 8 hours. She (or he) will not wait for your insurer to reimburse you. And please note that there is always the possibility that you won't be reimbursed. But I still think private nursing is a very worthwhile out-of-pocket expense, if you can afford it. So, determine ahead of time if you'll need to pay with personal checks or if the nursing office will take a credit card.

Scheduling

Obviously you will need to discuss timing of your surgery and absence with your boss, but don't forget to also talk with your spouse, life partner, and

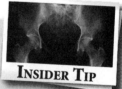

Avoid Scheduling Your Surgery For July or August

INSIDER TIP

July brings the new crop of interns and residents into the hospital, just in time for the bulk of surgeons to think about getting away this month or perhaps in August. These new doctors may know a lot about surgery, or they may be planning a career in psychiatry and are simply required to do a year of clinical medicine. Is this the best help available while you're at your most vulnerable? In addition, July and August are hot months and are just the time the AC in the hospital goes on the fritz, or the aides show up frazzled by the outside heat wave.

Workplace Considerations

It might be obvious, but if you're employed, you need to speak to the powers that be about the timing of your procedure, your absence, and the provisions for a medical leave of absence. Below are a few items to think about:

Out-of-work time: The average out-of-work time for a total hip replacement is 6 to 12 weeks. This span allows for differences in physical demand, age, associated medical problems, difficulty of transportation, among other factors. Lost work time may be considerably less after a hip resurfacing, but it may not. I have known some Resurf patients who are back at work within two weeks, while others have needed the full THR recovery time. Make sure that your surgeon agrees with your plan for returning to work and other activities.

Self-employment: If you're self-employed, you can still "speak to the boss" about what assignments you may not be able to cover for the first few weeks. But still, a little pre-planning never hurts.

other important people in your life who will be affected.

For the older patient, or one who has other arthritic or significant medical problems, winter is perhaps the least optimal time to schedule surgery. This is stating the obvious, but consider snow, ice, and transportation.

Information and Research

If your surgeon has a THR or Resurf video, make an appointment to see it. If you're squeamish, do ask first how graphic it is. It doesn't entirely substitute for a good verbal or written explanation, but it can be helpful.

	Surgical/ Anesthesia	Private Room/ Nurse	Physical Therapy
Medicare	All but 20 percent	No	Limited
HMO	All	No	Very limited
Medicaid	All	No	Very limited
Major Medical	All	Yes	Yes, at home and as long as you need

Home-Aide Equipment

This can be arranged through your social service representative in the hospital prior to discharge.

Costs and Coverage

Medicare may pay for a homemaker for a limited time and transportation to the physical therapy (PT) facility. You should call your insurer and find out exactly what they pay for, how long they pay for it, and what percentage you may be responsible for. What are the limits of their responsibility for transportation, rehabilitation, home aides, equipment, and how long a term do they cover?

I know extracting this information is not always simple, but get it now rather than trying to catch up after the fact. Also, try to get confirmation of coverage in writing. When you call, get the name and extension of the person you have spoken to, and the next time you call, ask for this same person. Otherwise you will always be starting from ground zero.

Chapter Seven Highlights

- Lose weight if you need to, exercise, and get a second opinion.
- Prepare your home and job for your post-op limitations.
- Don't forget about your pets.

Your Space

_____

_____

_____

_____

_____

_____

_____

_____

_____

_____

_____

_____

_____

_____

_____

_____

Prepare Your Nest

You would do well to consider your home, as it currently exists (pre-operatively), to be an obstacle course, totally unsuited to the returning post-op hero. If you have a spouse, partner, or live-in friend, you have an invaluable ally and protector, but you should still take some steps to make your recovery time at home easier and safer.

I am going to write these next paragraphs as if you have no one to help except a possible home-aide, you live in a three-story home, and you don't have an even semi-sedentary job. Many of these suggestions may be obvious, but you would still be wise to think about them all, and try to identify any other potential hazards you should fix that aren't listed here. Have your partner or care-giving friend read this as well.

"Hip-Proof" the House

If you've always thought of your home (apartment, condo, pad, or estate, etc.) as your safe nest, you're going to need to rethink this notion. In point of fact for post-op patients their home is full of traps and hazards.

House

- Take up all loose rugs.
- Make clear pathways from bed to front door, bathroom to kitchen, etc.
- Raise your bed on blocks, or arrange for a hospital bed to be delivered.
- Raise your favorite chair somewhere near the TV, or arrange to rent a high-seat chair.
- Put a table in the hall for newspaper/mail; you don't want to stoop or squat to get them.
- If you can, install handrails in shower and near toilet.
- Put non-slip mats in shower or bath tub.
- Have a cell phone or hands-free phone ready for use at all times.
- Place all pots and pans, dish-washing supplies, etc. to waist height—the lower

Sequential Thinking

INSIDER TIP

Most of us are used to planning—to some extent—our social calendar, our work projects, our vacations, etc., etc., etc.

But when it comes to a venture such as a THR or Resurf, we may not be as resourceful or see the benefit of planning. This is unfortunate, as one of the better things you can do for yourself is to keep track of exactly where you and your "keepers" are.

If you use the charts in Chapter Sixteen as you go through the other chapters, you will find you really grasp the event spectrum—from your procedure to your recovery.

Use the charts sequentially, and you may find you've developed the kind of sequential thinking your surgeon uses.

As one proverb has it: "A wise man is strong"; I would add "and smart!"

shelves in your kitchen, oven, and refrigerator are all forbidden territory.

- Clean house as thoroughly as possible.

Housekeeping

- Be sure that medications are near the sink, easy to reach, and have at least a three-week supply on hand.
- Stock lots of frozen food.
- Arrange clothes and cardigan sweaters, loafers or slip-on shoes where you can get them easily.
- Make sure you have at least one week's worth of pet food. Also arrange your pet's food and water dish above floor level (they'll get to it one way or another). Normal pet-care responsibilities must be given to a friend, partner, dog walker, or whomever—not you—for at least six weeks.
- Stop newspaper delivery during your hospitalization, or have a friend pick them up along with the mail.
- Arrange banking so that you (or partner) have access to cash for three weeks after your release from the hospital.
- Get a backpack for toting things around (frees your hands).

Also, Don't Forget . . .

- Make an emergency phone call list that includes your surgeon, M.D., siblings, physical therapist, home aide, etc. Keep this list close at hand, as you will need these numbers.
- Do not take anything beyond a few dollars to the hospital, much less any significant jewelry. Hospitals are notorious for their ability to absorb, misplace, and generally lose just about anything.
- Make a payback deal with your friend or partner (a bottle of champagne, a meal at his or her favorite restaurant, a trip to the South Pacific, a sable coat . . . you get the idea). Seriously, you will need help with things you couldn't imagine for the first weeks you're home.

To-Do List: 6 to 8 Weeks Prior to Surgery

As time moves on you need to think about specific time related pre-surgical actions and or plans.

Arrange for a Morning Surgery Time

Ask your surgeon to book a time slot as early in the day as possible on the surgical schedule. Your surgeon may be used to working all day, but the staff is fresher and more alert first thing in the morning. I've seen things go poorly—or at least more slowly—as the day goes by. If your surgery can be done in one-and-a-half hours in the am, the procedure may go as long as three hours near the end of the day. This is not to your advantage, and it also may add an extra hospital day to your stay.

Start Arranging Absence from Work

Inform all who must know, and help arrange your coverage. The coverage period you want to discuss is about six to eight weeks if your work is mostly sedentary and easily reached from your home. If you are a traveler or your work demands more in the way of physicality, you may want to count on 10 to 12 weeks. If you can do a lot from home, you can figure more in the area of three to four weeks.

Safe Car Driving with an Automatic Shift

Since you will be unable to drive following your surgery, you should make advance transportation arrangements. You should not plan to drive before 8 weeks minimum—and preferably 10 weeks—after you leave the hospital. If you have a stick shift, get a ride and don't even think about driving your car for a minimum of 12 to 16 weeks. It's not that you may not be able to manage the mechanics of driving, but rather that you may not be in full control in heavy traffic or if you need to stop suddenly. Imagine needing to make a quick stop at the exact moment that your hip misbehaves. God forbid you get into an accident while driving. As a recent hip recipient (less than 8 to 10 weeks), you won't have a legal leg to stand on (pun intended).

Minor Surgical and Dental Procedures

This is the time to get to the dentist for any necessary cleaning, or caps, or any oral surgery or procedure. This is also the time for any routine gynecology, proctology, or other routine exams. Even lesser cosmetic surgical procedures should be gotten out of the way. And, don't forget any serious things such as heart pacemaker adjustments or new batteries or whatever.

Arrange House and Pet Sitting

You can count on being in the hospital for five to six days, but it will be another six weeks until you're able to feed and water things and at least two to three months before you're ready to walk your dog. Enlist family, good friends or neighbors, or significant others for the period of your surgery and early convalescence. This is the time to begin arranging and coordinating it all.

Appointment to Pre-Donate Blood

You won't actually pre-donate until about one week to a few days before surgery, but now is when you should find out exactly where to go, the hours, and the procedures required to do so.

To-Do List: 2 to 3 Weeks Prior to Surgery

"As the time winds to a precious few," one needs to consider the following.

- Complete the blood donation arrangement.
- Check on private nursing arrangement, if you've made one.
- Talk to admitting office about your accommodation.
- State your preference regarding two-bedded, four-bedded, private room, or open ward. You can and should state a

preference and make a reservation, especially if you want a private room. Give the hospital a chance to arrange it for you. Demands or emergencies at the hospital may end up canceling your arrangements, so when you call it's not quite like making a confirmed hotel reservation. But, by and large, the admitting office will do its best.

- Finalize home and work arrangements.
- Change blood thinners (if you're taking them) two to three weeks before surgery, exactly as your internist has directed.
- Stop taking anti-inflammatory medication at least two weeks prior to surgery. You can switch to a medication that won't interfere with your blood clotting or coagulation (e.g., Tylenol). If you fail to do this, you could end up losing a great deal more blood on the operating table than you need. This is a risk you don't want to chance, even having reserved some of your own blood. You will also likely need a short-acting anticoagulant substance, such as some form and dosage of heparin. *Note:* Tylenol Extra-strength and Tylenol with codeine were of great help to me during this non-usual-anti-inflammatory medication period. They acted to lessen my pain and didn't interfere with clotting in the way many, if not most, anti-inflammatories do. I also used these two medications when I went to oral pain medication post-op.
- Report immediately to your surgeon *any* infections, either general or local (anything from a urinary tract infection or gall bladder attack to a boil, rash, or skin breakdown).
- Report immediately to your surgeon any change in your general medical status.
- Talk to both your anesthesiologist and internist about your long-term medical regimen and what to do about it for the last few weeks before surgery and *especially the day of surgery*. I'm talking about heart and blood pressure medications, insulin, or hormones of any sort, and any other regularly taken meds. Get specific and *written* instructions,

and be sure you understand them to the letter. (*Warning:* Surgeries have had to be canceled due to misunderstandings in this area. It is critical to your anesthesiologist and therefore to you.)

I know all of this may seem like a great deal of arranging to do when you don't feel in top form, but it will really pay off in terms of later peace of mind. Having all these details out of the way will leave you free to concentrate upon the most important things after surgery—your physical rehabilitation and re-adjustment.

To-Do List: 1 Week Prior to Surgery

I hesitate to call this the home stretch, but here we go.

Your "Take to Hospital" List

- Loafers or sandals. The hospital supplies slippers, but you will also need shoes that are very easy to put on for post-op rehab.
- Drawstring or loose, wide-bottom pants. My advice is buy a set at least two sizes larger than your normal. You'll need to get them over dressings and tubes easily.
- A cardigan-type sweater. Sometimes it's colder than you'd like when you're sitting in bed, a chair, or even in the corridors.
- Two loose shirts or large T-shirts. A change is nice.
- Two or more knee-high stockings/socks (keep warmth and comfort in mind).
- A robe of your own, unless you love hospital stripes and hit-or-miss fit. Bring your favorite nightgown or nightshirt, by all means. Forget pajamas—you won't be able to get in or out of them easily.

Note: For the first two days you may want to stay with standard-issue hospital gowns (the ones that give easy access to all parts of your body) because there will be many activities by the staff in the immediate post-op period that this garb facilitates. Afterward, when you again care what you look like, or are ready for public corridors, it's a different story.

- Basic toiletries. If you forget something, most basics are available from the hospital, but it's nicer if you have your own familiar things.
- Don't worry about the fine points of make-up, perfume, after-shave, etc. for the first two days. But be sure to include a comb and brush among the necessaries.
- Disposable pens, at least two (there will be forms to be signed, dietary check-off sheets, etc.).
- A credit card (TV deposit, and some go-home equipment may require it).
- A small amount of cash (for newspapers, etc.), no more than $20.
- If your first question on arriving at your bed will be "Where is my TV?" call Admitting as they will have all the answers for you.

Additional Advisable Items to Bring Along

- Paperback books. Don't bring heavy hardbacks; they can be awkward to hold. My suggestion is light reading or mysteries.
- Pre-stamped postcards or envelopes, pre-stuffed with sta-tionary. You may wish to write your friends from the hospital, and not worry over the details of how to.
- A *TV Guide* for the week, if you're a regular viewer.
- A small portable radio or iPod (consider bringing ear-phones for those times when others may not wish to listen to your programs).
- Telephone-address book. Not the encyclopedic one at home, but a small one with essential numbers of friends, relatives, doctors, important service providers you may need to be in touch with, etc.

- A notebook or writing pad for jotting reminders for your doctors, visiting friends, or whomever.
- By all means, a laptop, iPad, iPhone, or its like if you're Cyber cathected.
- Transportation home from the hospital—a cab service, an accommodating friend, or a relative with a "decent-size" car.

The Night Before Surgery

If you have developed any infection, no matter how general or local (anything from a urinary tract infection or gallbladder flare-up to a boil, rash, or skin lesion), you must report this immediately to your surgeon. Any of these may cause your surgery to be canceled—for your own protection.

You must also report any change in your general medical status, such as diabetic control problem, fever of any kind, or any cold or flu symptoms, as this may also result in cancellation of your surgery.

Here are a few night-before to-dos:

- *Pack your copy of this book.*
- Lay out your clothes.
- Clip your toenails.
- Take nothing by mouth after midnight—not even water if you can help it.
- Above all, take no pills that are not sanctioned by your internist, your surgeon, or the anesthesiologist!
- You might think to say a little blessing for your surgical team, having said one already for yourself.

If you arrange to cover most of the things in this chapter, you should have the sense of doing everything in your power to help yourself, which is a good feeling when you're about to undergo surgery, which is entirely in someone else's hands.

Chapter Eight Highlights

- Hip-proof your house.
- Get medical clearance for surgery and check medications.
- Prepare for a hospital stay of three to five days.

Your Space

_____

_____

_____

_____

_____

_____

_____

_____

_____

_____

_____

_____

_____

_____

In the Hospital–
Before and After
Surgery

This is a day that may begin somewhere between annoyance, regret, or panic, and end in complete oblivion. All told, it will be a strange 24-hour period in your life. It rolls on with little you can do to speed or impair it, and you may remember only a few of the specifics afterwards.

The beginning of your day consists of waiting. The admitting office will have you wait, then ask you for signatures, then you'll wait and give more signatures, and finally wait again as you're being processed through.

Ultimately, when you get to the surgical floor, you will wait yet again as you slowly go through the pre-surgical holding area, and then—at least if you experience the average day of surgery—you'll wait still before being taken into the operating room. This isn't easy on the patient who's keyed up for surgery, but by and large it's the way things happen. The important thing to bear in mind is that your surgery *will happen*.

Admission

Most patients come in as same-day patients, meaning they are checked in on the same day surgery is planned—an efficiency instituted by insurance companies. If you have a calm and steady member of the family, bring him or her with you at check-in for support, and for any last-minute instructions you may wish to give. If you have only nervous Nellies, you should insist they stay home, and brave the admitting office on your own. In any case, when the aide comes to take you to the surgical floor, visitors of any kind have got to leave.

Your admission to the hospital via the admitting office is routine. In prepping you for the "admissions process," I want you to know that, by and large, admitting is staffed by a group whose primary responsibility is to get the massive paperwork done, and done right. Don't expect or demand personal consideration or humor. Do anticipate impatience, non-communication, and a focus on numerous forms. Going in with these expectations will serve you well—even if your admitting clerk is one of the rare ones who actually sees the patient behind the admitting process. Remember, their primary responsibility is admissions, and my suggestion that you anticipate this is only intended to help you avoid stress.

So, be prepared to handle the mechanics and processing outlook of the admitting office—don't get angry and try not to take it personally; it isn't meant that way.

Sign everything on demand if the major headings are accurate (e.g., type and site of surgery, insurance company, doctors). If you are having a difficult time reading the small print, please ask for help or have your companion help with these important documents. The object is to get this part of your day over with as soon as you can. Remind admitting again of your room arrangements. It gives you a better shot at actually getting them.

Ultimately, you will be put in a wheelchair and taken to the preoperative prep and holding area. No, the hospital can't permit you to walk, even if you're capable—this is a "medico-legal" issue.

Pre-Operative Holding Area

The pre-op holding area is where you will be required to make the transition from person and patient. It's pretty unavoidable, so go with the flow. This transition includes:

- Street clothes to a unisex hospital gown with little choice of size (and Dior it ain't). Hospital gowns are designed first for access and second to expose, not cover.
- Plastic wrist ID band with your assigned hospital number printed in large type, and your name—often misspelled—in lesser type. The staff will check your ID over and over with it, often to look up each time and say your name aloud with a question mark.
- Repeated basic questions, ranging from who's your doctor to what you're going to have done, often while reading from a form that already states most of the info. *Be patient.*
- Above all, **be sure to answer any and all questions about allergies**, no matter how often they're asked.
- You are then strapped down to a stretcher (the official name is gurney). And no matter what it's called, it's your operating room transit vehicle.
- An IV line is put in your arm. (This can be slightly painful.)
- Again, you'll sign multiple consent forms for the hospital, anesthesiologist, your MD, etc. This may take a while, and when it's all completed you may still stay in the holding area for an hour or two, again *waiting.*

The Operating Room

So finally, you're wheeled into the operating room (O.R.) and transferred to the operating table. The transfer for a THR candidate can be painful, awkward, and slow. You may glimpse equipment, hear the sound of metal on metal, see people in various get-ups coming in and going out of the room, and there is a distinct smell to an O.R., all quite alien even if you've had surgery before. The chances are that, post-op, you will remember none of the details. But this is the way it should be.

Anesthesia

The anesthesia process starts with some form of sedation, so you can hear and cooperate when needed, but you'll feel like you're in la-la land, which is where your surgeon wants you. You'll have had an IV started, and it's through this that you'll receive the sedation.

As mentioned earlier, the anesthesia of choice for a THR is called a continuous epidural. At this point, either your surgeon or your anesthesiologist will tell you how it's done.

You will be asked to flex and curl your back to the best of your ability. A tiny bore catheter is inserted into the outer layer of your spinal canal. Medication (often a substance called Bipucaine) is given through this catheter, taking all sensation away below the level of insertion, but leaving you the ability to move. The catheter is then inserted to administer the anesthetic; it will be left in place for some period post-op. It is a perfect regional pain controller. An epidural has the added advantage of helping to moderate high blood pressure, for those patients who have this medical condition. It is the *kindest* type of anesthesia, and it can be left in place and going for the first 48 to 60 hours post-op. You can move, even stand, wiggle your toes, and move about in bed, but you'll feel no pain and won't be "zonked."

Only if a spinal catheter can't be placed for anatomical reasons will general anesthesia be considered, at least in most of the United States. Elsewhere in the world, they may be able to do a continuous epidural, but you may have to battle it out with anesthesiologists who are more accustomed to giving a "general"—essentially gas.

In the view of most U.S.-trained anesthesiologists who are accustomed to doing THRs, the safest method is an epidural. Some things we get very right, and continuous epidural is one of them. In any case, you will also be given a sedative that may knock you out for at least the duration of the procedure, and through your stay in the recovery room.

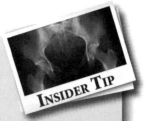

Things to Keep in Mind in the Prep Room

INSIDER TIP

With all the activity and conversation going on around you, you may feel small and unimportant, and in alien territory. You may be made to feel that in a sense you're part of the problem, due to all the commotion of a functioning O.R. But, without you and others around you, there'd be no need to open the O.R. this day.

- This is the time to remind the operating room staff of your pre-donated blood.
- If you're cold, there are extra blankets available if you ask, and if you'd like a sip of water via ice chips, that's doable as well.
- I've had patients who seemed to like looking around at the general activity and others who closed their eyes waiting quietly with their own thoughts for their turn. I took a duplicate mystery story and read in between answering questions. (Duplicate because there's every chance the book may not find its way to your room, other things being more important in the immediate post-op period). Again, in all likelihood you'll remember little of this time.
- Even if you don't see your surgeon in the "prep room" prior to surgery, I promise you he will see you in the O.R.
- In some hospitals, the anesthesiologist will start an IV drip here in the prep room.

Immediately After Surgery

In some hospitals, and depending somewhat on your general medical condition, you may be kept overnight in the recovery room or even the Intensive Care Unit. The level of monitoring possible on the regular hospital floor may not be sufficient for the immediate post-op period. If all systems are go after 6 to 10 hours of monitoring with vital signs and condition remaining stable, you'll be transported to your room.

The day of surgery is a time for you to have faith in the wisdom of your decision, the care of the hospital staff, and the skill of your surgeon. You will have little to no recollection of most of the events after your anesthesiologist gives you sedation, no matter how vividly you may later recall the admissions office experience.

Chapter Nine Highlights

- Hospital admission may be the hardest part.
- You *must* communicate to staff every and all allergies.
- In the O.R., go with the flow. The team knows what they are doing.

Your Space

_____

_____

_____

_____

_____

_____

_____

_____

_____

_____

_____

_____

_____

_____

_____

_____

The First Day

For those of you who've had a Resurf rather than a THR, you'll find this chapter to be of some interest, but even more to the point is Chapter Eleven, which discusses days two through five.

In the beginning (day one post-op) you may feel pretty helpless, bed-bound, and as if you've been run over by a Mack truck. You're entitled to feel tired. Your body has been through a lot, even if you were not aware of it at the time it happened. But, quite remarkably, by day four, if you're the usual patient, you will have cabin fever, having felt confined too long to the hospital and its routines.

Expect that this patient-to-person transition starts on day two or three post-op. Day one is the period when you discover that you have survived. Your pain is controllable. You are being monitored closely, you're full of "lines" and equipment, and you're relatively comfortable in bed.

Identifying Tubes or Lines

- Your IV line, in your hand or arm, is taped in securely. Antibiotics, fluids, and anticoagulants are given via this line; all comes under the heading of fluid input.

- Your antibiotic, run in over time, is piggy-backed into your IV.
- A Foley catheter was inserted into your bladder while you were on the operating table. This serves to measure part of your fluid output.
- Drains, at least one, from your surgical site, emerge from under your dressing and are another critical fluid output measuring device. They also serve to drain away fluid so that it does not accumulate deep within your surgical wound.
- Fluid balance is critical to your well-being. Your medical team is particularly concerned about build-up or accumulation of fluids that might accumulate in your lungs and/or produce swelling in your legs, both of which are highly undesirable; hence the careful measurement of input/output.
- You may still have the epidural (spinal) line in place. Piggy-backed in this line is your patient-controlled pain medication. If you have any trouble with it, your nurse will monitor and use it for you, or help you do so. A limit is set on how much you may select, allowing a sufficient amount to take care of your pain, but not enough to cause an overdose.

Identifying Other Equipment

- An abduction splint or pillow maintaining a critical abduction (legs wide-apart) position. You will learn over the next few weeks that this position is an essential one for post THRs. You will become, rightfully, super aware of it. It *prevents dislocations.*
- Elastic knee-high stockings or the more desirable sequential compression device (SCD), an automatic device which inflates and deflates rhythmically, pumping your calves, encouraging circulation within your legs. Both are anti-clot-forming aids.

I far prefer the pneumatic anti-embolic device (SCD), which is state of the art for preventing calf clots or thrombi, which are one of the premier first week's risks or hazards. It is an active, more specific approach to the problem of venous stasis—the pooling of blood in your legs when you are immobile—that in turn encourages clot formation.

- Most hospital beds come with an overhead trapeze, to help you in turning and getting out of bed. Also, anticipate side-rails on your bed, which the staff will insist must be up at all times except when you're getting out of bed. This is a slight inconvenience, but protective.

Inhalation Spirometer

You must learn and master the blow bag, or inhalation spirometer. A nurse or aide will demonstrate how to use it. I strongly suggest you give it a go six or eight times during the first 24 hours. It is something useful you can do on your own behalf to protect yourself against post-op pulmonary problems.

First-Day Activities

The resident doctors (part of the hospital staff) will see you during their rounds early on your first post-op morning, usually between 5:30 and 7 am. This is done to assess your general condition, the state of your input/output, and other vital statistics (blood pressure, pulse, temperature), and whether all your tubes and attachments are functioning correctly. All will be recorded in your chart. The chart thus becomes an important physical evaluation tool for all who will care for you.

At around 7 am, a nurse will visit you and check your blood pressure, pulse, temperature, and output measurements. You can expect return nursing visits and procedures in the evening.

Breakfast will be between 7:30 and 8 am, lunch between 11:30 am and noon, and dinner between 5:30 and 6 pm. If you're not hungry, kindly send the tray away, and don't worry—

you will survive. The critical thing for the first day or so is that you *drink* clear fluids.

My suggestion is that you pick light and simple things to eat during your stay, as your digestive system will handle them better. If you are given a check-off list, select from that; if not, pick and choose from the plate you are offered. The dietitian should come to talk with you. If you need kosher, vegetarian, or hypoallergenic food, tell her, and the kitchen will do its best to accommodate. However, gourmet cooking is probably not in the cards.

Your surgeon may appear to check you over at any time this first day, depending on his schedule, as will your internist. Your anesthesiologist or some-

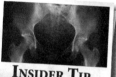

INSIDER TIP

If You Think Something Is Wrong . . . Speak Up!

None of the tubes should cause you pain! If they do, you must let someone know. For example, the IV in your hand or arm can slip out of its proper place in the vein and infiltrate the soft tissues around it. This results in local swelling and/or pain. If your IV begins to hurt, call for immediate attention. However you have to get attention—get it. The problem should be attended to as soon as possible. The reasons, I think, are obvious.

In the self-help department, you are the first person who can pick up on a medical problem that will help your medical team. No one but you can determine if your IV, or catheter, or drain is causing pain—only you. Any of these will then need attention.

You will have a call bell, usually at eye level and to your right. This rings at the central nursing station of your floor and will summon help, soon or late, depending on what else is happening on the floor at the time.

one from the anesthesiology department will also visit. Discuss pain control. Be sure you have a good level of pain relief, because you get no points for heroism. Talk over how long the epidural line may be left in place. My suggestion is that you ask for it to be left to cover pain through post-op day two. It can be removed after your physical therapy session on that second day.

Your blood will be tested many times, for indications of excessive blood loss, electrolyte imbalance, and early signs of infection. Be prepared to be stuck with a needle more often in the next day or two than you have in the last few months (see "Getting Through the Needle Sticks"). It's a routine post-op procedure and monitoring. However, it can be slightly painful.

Getting Through the Needle Sticks

You are at the mercy of a special technician who does nothing else from dawn to dusk except draw blood. If he or she is new on the job, you may be in for a couple of misses. If your technician is an old pro, the process is quick and with minimal pain.

After a day or two of veni-punctures (needle sticks), you may acquire a good-sized black and blue spot, either on the inside of your elbow or the back of your hand. This bruise can be tender. It is usually the result of small, fragile veins leaking slightly after being punctured. Ask your nurse for warm compresses and a little topical benzocaine.

It's a good idea to ask the tech to vary sides and sites. Try not to yelp or move when being stuck—it may lead to the tech causing you even more pain. In any case, put up with it as best you can, because blood test results are just as important as monitoring your blood pressure or temperature.

This is the day that—despite all your attached equipment—you will be gotten out of bed and into a chair (specifically a high-seated chair) for at least one hour. Occupational and physical therapists will visit you for the first time, and may leave a walker by your bedside. Physical therapy (P.T.) will see to rehabilitating your muscles and walking. Occupational therapy (O.T.) will supervise learning new techniques for activities of daily living.

Generally speaking, the hospital staff and your occupational and physical therapists know what they're doing. They've seen and dealt with dozens—if not hundreds—of "post-THRs" and Resurfs, in all kinds of physical and medical conditions. If you give them your input (e.g., what's difficult, what's easy; which maneuvers hurt, which don't; when you're tired, when you can go one more round), they will be able to tailor their skill to your individual needs.

Note: You don't have to be in love with an individual staff member (resident, nurse, aide, physical therapist, or occupational therapist worker), but you do want to get the most from their skills and experience. So ask for what you need to know or use, and let most of the complaints about personality and charm go for when you are out of the hospital (and their reach) and you are recounting your "horrendous" experience to a circle of sympathetic friends.

Ask for Pain Medication if You Need It

Don't hesitate to ask for or use pain medication during the first 48 hours post-op, after surgery. It's okay. Pain from the amount of surgery done to your body is expected; it doesn't arise from the actual hip prosthesis. Remember that installing your new hip required all of the muscles and subcutaneous tissues on the way in to be manipulated, and they may now let you know about it.

Don't be a stoic and let pain go until it becomes severe. It's much easier to deal with and needs much less analgesics to

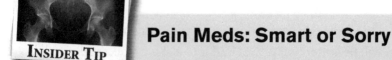
Pain Meds: Smart or Sorry

Everyone associated with your surgery wants your pain to be controlled, especially for the first few days. It's possible that you are one of the fortunate few who have very little pain, but if not, help your doctors to help you.

- There is a trick to pain management. Catch it early and you control it better with less medication.
- If you wait until the pain is full-blown, you evoke full-blown opiate measures and a zonked state.
- There are no points to be gained by being stoic about the matter. Your doctors, the nurses, and the hospital personnel all know pain is expected as a part of post-op-ness.

control when still mild. The floor resident can prescribe something like Tylenol for mild pain within a short time, if your surgeon has not included this in his or her orders.

Dislocations

Make every effort not to turn or twist in bed. Get used to sleeping on your back for a while in order to avoid dislocating your new hip. Train yourself to accept the abduction pillow and pneumatic anti-embolic stockings virtually 24 hours a day. It's not as hard as you think if you make up your mind.

Getting Nursing Help

Floor nurses and /or aides are very hard to get during certain times:

- Shift changes, which are generally 7:30 am and 7:30 pm.

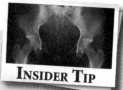
- When medications or meals are being served.
- When new patients are coming to the floor from surgery.
- If the nursing supervisory personnel come to visit.
- If there's an emergency on the floor.

For those of you who can do so, having a private nurse makes a significant difference, especially during the day shifts (8 am to 4 pm).

It may sound idiotic, but be sure you know where your bedside buzzer (call bell) is at all times, and exactly how it works. If you need help in a hurry, the buzzer may not produce it, so don't hesitate to enlist one of your more mobile roommates to go and get someone.

Sleep this first night may come easily. If it doesn't, ask for sleeping medication. Your doctor has prescribed something to help you sleep, should you need it.

Don't Worry About Feeling a Bit Disoriented

You will remember little if anything at all about the day of surgery. But you also may have slight problems with present orientation and memory, in the form of slight memory lapses, a general fuzziness, or a sense of drifting in and out of full awareness for the first 24 to 36 hours after surgery. Do not worry; this feeling will pass before day two or three post-op.

Major surgery plus the uprooting experience of being in a hospital is a real glitch in the flow of your mental life. I am convinced that sedation and anesthesia sufficient to carry you through the procedure itself almost always produces after-effects. The exact effect varies by individual. You may struggle to remember names and events, or you just don't feel really "sharp" the first few days after surgery, or perhaps you need your nurses and therapists to repeat information or instructions. Maybe you won't recall something your surgeon said or described. It's okay; be a little patient with yourself. Don't anticipate this to be a permanent condition.

Anti-P.E. (Pulmonary Embolism)

You will receive an anti-coagulant (or anti-clotting) medication to discourage thrombus formation. Exactly which medication is prescribed will be the result of your surgeon's experience and judgment, and there is no medical unanimity on just which one is best. There is also no strict unanimity on how long after surgery you should receive this medication. If you have been on such medication pre-operatively, you will be restored as quickly as possible to your old regimen.

On one thing there is complete medical agreement: Early mobilization and activity are essential for your circulation and respiration and general condition. So go with the flow—up and out of bed as soon and as often as possible.

And so to bed; the first day is behind you. Bravo!

Chapter Ten Highlights

- You will wake up to tubes you never imagined—each one necessary.
- Abduction device to prevent dislocation—an essential treatment.
- First day as a blur is normal; not to worry.

Your Space

Days Two through Five

Between days two and five, you'll start to make the transition back from patient to person. There are a couple of things to bear in mind. Days two through five will be full of activities and learning—and probably visitors, especially those friends and relatives who've seen or been through some of your pre-operative problems.

Visitors

In general, visitors have a tendency to over-stay. It's hard to convince them that 15 to 20 minutes can get it all done. If possible, delegate your nearest and dearest to tell them of visiting hours, and to encourage them to keep their visit short so as not to over-tire you, especially post-op day two.

Try to have your visiting delegate limit the number of people in the room at any one time. It is tiring to "entertain" many people at once. If you are not in a private room, your neighboring bedfellows will thank you.

Back to diet for a moment . . . unlike those who have undergone surgery for other reasons, an orthopedic patient has options. You don't have to force down the blue-plate special of the day. Assuming your doctor has no objections, use your friends to visit your favorite deli or gourmet shop. Even frozen foods can be heated up. There's a microwave at every nursing station for the staff to use. If you ask nicely, they'll probably nuke yours too, or at least let you do so.

Visiting hours are set the way they are in order to clear the floor when the nursing and other staff have duties to perform that visitors would interfere with. If it is vital that you see someone whose schedule doesn't permit them to visit you during regular visiting hours, talk to either your doctor or the nursing supervisor for your floor. One of them may be able to arrange another time.

If you wind up with too many flowers, send the older ones to the nursing station for the staff to give out. There are many patients on the floor who get none and would be grateful.

Physical Therapy

It is wise to remember that everyone recuperates from THR or a Resurf at different rates. The features and characters of a physical therapy program vary. Do not compare your activities to those of another THR patient. Do not get discouraged if a given activity comes to you more slowly than it did for someone else.

If you want evaluation of your progress, ask your therapist how you are progressing. You will get the most authoritative and apt response.

As for the in-hospital P.T. facility, I've seen everything from an overgrown equipment closet to an entire floor. Suffice it to say that physical therapists, as a group, are among the most inventive and encouraging of experts. Most, if not all, believe totally in what they're doing and in what you can achieve. They will educate as well as inspire you.

Do remember to give them feedback, so that your program really fits you and progresses you to the maximum. They will start off with a general idea of what you should be doing and how often. Let them tailor it to your abilities.

Be sure to ask for a series of exercises you can do on your own in bed to help you build muscle tone. Doing these at least twice a day, both in bed or in a chair, augments your P.T. program and puts you way ahead in general recuperation. Ask to be taught these exercises for bed use:

- Isometric quads.
- Buttock squeezes.
- Pelvic tilts.
- Gastroc flexion/extension (squeezes).
- Ankle motion.

Your therapist will know these exercises and can help you with them. Starting with day three, ask for two P.T. sessions per day, if that can be arranged.

Also on day three, you should begin to be able to get out of bed on your own and slowly start walking, even a few steps, either with a walkerette or with crutches.

The Transition from IV to Oral Medication

You will continue to need antibiotics, a blood-thinner, and pain medication. On day three, assuming your recovery is proceeding normally, your IV will be stopped and you'll go onto oral medication.

You may find that you need to take something for constipation, which is normal for post-op or sedentary conditions. Ask one of the resident staff who makes rounds to order something for you.

Ask to be given pain medication at the hours you need it rather than on the hospital's standard schedule. That way you'll be able to get an analgesic an hour before your P.T. sessions, and at night, when you may find you have most need of help. By the way, the increase in pain many experience at night is probably due to two things: You're paying for some of your daytime activities, and at night there are fewer distractions and, thus, more opportunity for awareness of pain.

Other Transitions

The main transition concerns the removal of various tubes or "lines."

- Removal of your epidural line is virtually painless.
- Removing your IV is at least quick. But you will feel it.
- Removal of the Foley catheter is more problematic, especially for men. For women, it's easier and produces a little pain and irritation. For men, however, with the catheter positioned as it is in the penis, it can be a bit more unpleasant. And the first or second urination may produce some burning, hesitation, or a few drops

About Bedpans

INSIDER TIP

I have always found one of the hardest things both athletically, and esthetically, to use is a bedpan. I simply can't do it, surrounded by curtains or not. For the first 48+ hours you will not need one. The Foley catheter takes care of urination, and you won't need to defecate during this time. After the first 48 hours, learn to use your walker well enough to get to a bathroom, as there will be one, either in your room or just next door in the corridor. If this is not possible, ask for a bedside commode, which you will find easier and safer to use than a bedpan.

of blood. If you know you have a prostate problem, talk to the resident staff or nurses about it, particularly if the Foley removal aggravates it. This may or may not occur, but if it does it's usually transitory and is not an unknown to the staff. If the problem continues, ask for a urologic consult.

Dressing changes, which start on day two or three and occur daily thereafter, are not a pleasure because the tape (usually plastic or treated paper) must be removed. In general, the area around your incision will be tender, swollen, and discolored if you're anywhere near average patient. This sense of tenderness and bruising may go on for a week or two. You may also feel a sense of pinching at the site of the sutures or staples. When the area is handled and inspected, expect some discomfort. It's inevitable.

Removal of the wound drainage tubes, which may take place anytime from day three to day four, is definitely not a joy. The lines are usually secured in place with a stitch that must be cut, and the actual tug and sensation of the line being withdrawn from inside is painful. Fortunately this is not a prolonged procedure, and your surgeon or surgical staff who does it knows it hurts and tries to be quick.

Washing is a pleasure with a private nurse, who will follow it with back rubs or light massage. Otherwise, here are a few suggestions for the first few days in the bed bath department:

- Be sure you're steady with your walker before attempting a shower.
- Pre-plan a back-pack arrangement; it works well for soap, shampoo, toweling, talc, etc.
- After day two, shaving seems to make men feel more human, and some minor cosmetics seems to do the same for women.
- Switch to your own robe and/or clothing; don't stay in hospital wear. Change is good for your morale, as is the feeling of becoming your own person again, even in the hospital setting.

Activities of Daily Living

No matter what it takes in terms of your effort, in spite of all your connected tubing, with much help from the staff, you will be gotten up out of bed and placed in a chair at least twice on day one after surgery.

You will be shown how to help move your legs *safely* to the edge of your bed, how to transfer to a walker, and then how to get from a standing position to a sitting one. It's a procedure that you will have to master as a new technique of activity or daily living. Be sure you know exactly how to get out of bed and onto your walker safely under supervision before you dream of doing this on your own. When you are seated for the first time upright in a chair:

- Be sure you know how to summon immediate help, before staff leaves you.
- If you feel at all dizzy or faint, say so at once; heroes get in trouble in hospitals.
- Not everyone can do the out-of-bed-into-chair routine *twice* on day two. It's okay to go at your pace, as long as you're aware of the need to try to push your activities a little.

In fact, you will have to relearn many activities that you took for granted from the point of view of *protecting your new hip against dislocation.* You will learn to have a special awareness of what you're doing and how you're doing it; it is an essential re-education. It's not that you should *fear* dislocating your hip during a given activity, but more that you need to think about what will be hazardous and pre-plan how to go about activities and transfers.

Awareness of Difficulty or Trouble

You may well be the first person to pick up early on a post-op problem, so be very aware of any of the following:

- Developing a cough or any difficulty in breathing.
- Calf pain.
- Increasing thigh or wound pain.
- Sweatiness or the feeling of excessive heat.
- Any lessening of your ability to do the post-op activities you were taught.

You must do something ASAP! Do not assume it's okay— IT'S NOT! Communicate it as soon as possible to your nurse or a resident doctor.

Coughing, difficulty breathing, or calf pain may be early signs of a pulmonary embolism or pneumonia. Either must be treated early and aggressively to arrest its progress. Increased pain, sweating, or lessening ability to do post-op activities may be early signs of a wound infection, which also needs diagnosis followed by quick and aggressive counteraction.

Post-Op Wound Infections

Post-op wound infections can occur, and there are two types to look out for.

Superficial: Those that are confined to the outer layers of the wound and may be treated locally with superficial opening and cleaning.

Deep: These are the ones that surgeons worry about. They involve infection of the inner layers of the surgical wound, the joint, and prosthesis. This type of infection, as noted, will probably involve a second visit to the O.R., general anesthesia, a thorough debridement (clean-out) of the deep tissues, and even removal of the prosthesis.

I cannot tell you exactly the course your surgeon will choose to treat a deep wound infection; it is a matter of what he finds and his judgment as to exactly what to do about it. About 40 percent of these infections respond favorably to debridement alone. Another 20 to 30 percent are able to have the prosthesis replaced after three to six weeks of antibiotics, with or sometimes without a second debridement.

Though there is no hard-and-fast consensus or protocol for treating a deep infection like this, the heart of it is debridement of infected tissue, taking a culture to determine which antibiotic to start, and wide drainage of the depths of the wound.

A deep infection is definitely a matter of serious concern, and that is why so many preventive measures are taken: the antibiotic coverage that started when you were on the operating table, the use of Laminar airflow and "spacesuits" in the O.R., and the antibiotic irrigation of your surgical site when open on the table.

The figures I quoted you for post-op wound infections are not written in stone, due to differing criteria of reporting. I have shared what are considered the higher-side figures. The point is for you to understand that some superficial infections, *if let go*, or treated late rather than early, can develop into deep infections. If you develop noticeable heat in your thigh, or increasing soreness and swelling, you should bring these to the attention of the resident staff or your surgeon as soon as possible. Hopefully they will take a look and tell you the amount of swelling, heat, or discomfort is acceptable, as I urge you to be overly cautious rather than miss early signs of an infection. The word for your guidance is *complain* when in thigh pain!

Bear in mind that more than 95 percent of THRs go smoothly without the slightest complication or difficulty. This compares favorably with other major surgical procedures. Now . . .

The "Rehab Floor"

In a larger hospital, sometime during your penultimate stay, usually the third day after surgery, it may be proposed that you move to the rehab floor (a step down from the intensive medical care you have had for the first 72 hours). Your answer to this proposition should be a decided *yes*! You'll be ready for this move. This is more than just a shift in locale, and more than a shift in focus; it is a change from acute medical care and attention to a more restorative, or recuperative, type of patient care. It requires you to be a participant in a program focused on physical activity. You will continue to be monitored medically, but with less intensity—it's really a kind of a halfway house. Therefore, be sure to pay attention to your own body's early warning signs. Continue to give feedback to your therapist so that your P.T. program progresses in the way that's best for you.

Take advantage of the practice this "halfway house" affords you. You're still harbored by the hospital setting, but you'll be free to set many of your own habits and work on ambulatory skills. Don't forget your in-bed exercises, especially calf-squeezing and buttock work.

You're ready somewhere around day three, the 48-hour-to-discharge landmark, to begin your hospital-to-home transition.

From Soup to Nuts

Before you go home:

- Have someone cut your toenails if you haven't done this before you came to the hospital.
- Have your hair shampooed. Your nurse will help with this.
- Be sure you have all the equipment for daily living that you were taught to use and arranged for in your possession, or home delivery confirmed.

Post-Op for Resurf Patients

By and large, the hospital stay may be a minimum of two to four days, even for you Resurf recipients. The immediate concerns about fluid balance, clot formation, wound care, and drainage are essentially the same, and just as serious.

However, there is far less concern about dislocations. You may be asked to keep the abduction pillow when in bed, but the rest of the time it is not necessary. There will be a far more aggressive push for getting you up and about, with almost full weight bearing. You are younger and in better health, by and large, than the average THR patient.

Low chairs are not such a problem. Moderate forward bending is possible. The return to normal activities is more rapid, limited primarily by how much local pain or discomfort you have in your thigh and buttock due to the surgery.

The concerns about embolic phenomenon are the same, and the medication for it as rigorous. Likewise is the concern for wound infections.

Your return-to-work dates will be much sooner, and limited only by how quickly your soft tissue responds to surgery. However, timing of suture or staple removal and wound care are the same as with THRs.

Unlike the typical THR, your Resurf hip may produce "squeaking" sounds that may start in the hospital. This phenomenon may lessen over time and be of no further consequence. If not, your surgeon will review it on a subsequent visit. "Clunking" on the other hand, may infer future troubles with your Resurf, but only time and careful following will determine if this is a big deal. Let your surgeon help interpret the sounds your hip is making.

Chapter Eleven Highlights

- Physical therapy is the most important step at this juncture.
- You are the first to be aware of unexplained difficulties or pain—speak up.
- Post-op for Resurfs may vary from THRs.

Your Space

_____

_____

_____

_____

_____

_____

_____

_____

_____

_____

_____

_____

_____

_____

_____

_____

_____

Before You Go Home

The last 48 hours in the hospital are busy, demanding days. If you're the usual patient you will probably feel pretty good because you've been through the worst and you have much less discomfort and much more mobility than when you came into the hospital. Your P.T. program has become more and more advanced, and you are becoming more and more independent. Life, in short, should be looking up for you, as it certainly did for me. But you have much to do before discharge.

Be sure that Occupational Therapy and Physical Therapy know as much as possible about your home situation!

Think about your steps inside and out, difficult doors, or placement of essential objects, bathing facilities, closets, storage spaces, etc. Think about it, and work out the odd and specific arrangements that may challenge you. Again, get a backpack to carry whatever you need so that you can open a sticky door on two crutches; it will be easier. By the way, try to carry your front door keys in an easy-to-get-to pocket or around the neck—even better.

Your Occupational Therapist and Your Social Worker

Two people will become very important helpers at this point. Let's start with the first one—your occupational therapist. Be sure he or she has introduced you to the following:

- The long-reach grasper, which permits you to reach and pick up objects you cannot stoop for and may help with dressing and positioning shoes.
- Stocking aid, which permits you to put on socks or stockings without hazard.
- Soap-on-a-rope. When you shower, it's always in reach.
- The high-seated chair.
- The raised, portable toilet seat.
- And, of course, your walker and crutches.

Your occupational therapist will tell you to buy the toilet seat, and sometimes the stocking aid and grabber. Often the hospital simply gives you the last two items. She'll then make arrangements for you to rent your walker, crutches, and a high chair. She also may concern herself with how you and your equipment will get home; or, this issue may be handled by your social worker.

That leads us to the second important person in your life, your social worker. He or she will be an amazing conduit of information and help, and is possibly the most key figure in your last two hospital days. Here are some of the problems I asked about; you may have others. Your therapist (O.T.) and your social worker will have the answers to many questions, some of which may be how much of the equipment is covered by your insurance, and how to arrange for home-making help, and whether insurance will cover it.

If your significant other can't help out with home-making chores, and you don't have a friend who can help out on a more-or-less regular basis, you will need an aide to help with shopping and cleaning for the first three to four weeks. Your social worker will arrange for this aide as well as the following:

Physical therapy at home: This is usually covered by insurance, and it may be your only official continuing physical therapy. It is also a good idea to use an outpatient center for continuing rehabilitation at least once or twice a week. Your social worker will make the arrangement, and will tell you how much outpatient therapy is covered by your insurance.

Visiting nurse service: A nurse should see you *at least once a week* for the first three to four weeks when you go home to keep an eye on your general condition, check your surgical site, and to assist with any medical problems or questions that may arise. Unfortunately, there still exists the possibility of post-surgical complications (these must be watched for). Infection and embolism can occur within the first three weeks and occasionally even months post surgery. Granted, this is not nearly as likely as in the first week or so, but it has been reported in medical literature. Many surgeons believe in continuing anti-coagulant therapy with low doses of aspirin for the first 6 to 12 weeks after surgery; I am one of them.

Appointments: Before you leave the hospital, where all your care was on a scheduled basis, you may feel more secure if you have a definite appointment time for each of the following: surgeon, internist, outpatient P.T. facility, home therapist, homemaker (if desired), and delivery of your high chair. Note the time, date, address, and telephone numbers on your calendar.

Now all the work you did preparing your nest will pay off. If by chance you didn't do this, get a good friend, partner, neighbor, or relative to read Chapter Eight about preparing your nest and setting up your home. The key to planning for your return home is to bear in mind the idea that you will be semi-independent for the next few weeks. And the other mantras are, as you've learned, awareness and pre-planning.

And so to bed, plans well laid, resources organized on your last night in the hospital.

Posthab Exercise

Post surgery, the goal of your exercise program should be to *gradually* restore normal hip motion and strength. Your orthopedic surgeon and physical therapist may recommend exercise for 20 to 30 minutes two or three times a day during early recovery. Do your best, and—again—if you feel pain, speak up immediately.

The post rehab process after total hip replacement occurs early in the post-operative period, actually within the first 6 to 8 weeks. You will typically start physical therapy the day after surgery to help you regain and improve strength around the operative hip.

The Issue of Post-Op Pain and Exercise

Very few among the sane of this world suffer absolutely *no* pain after a joint replacement or resurfacing. After all, someone did take a knife to your leg and cut through some pretty large muscles.

Pain is one of the most subjective experiences we must handle in life. There are those who can tolerate a lot, and those who are more pain sensitive.

- Fear intensifies pain.
- Anxiety about the unfamiliar intensifies pain.
- If the procedure you've just undergone was surgically complicated or took more than the usual manipulation and/or attention on the operating table, you are likely to have more pain.

However, by the time it is reasonable for a THR or Resurf patient to begin serious exercise, it should cause little actual pain, and certainly not in the hip joint. If it does, you must notify your surgeon.

With a total knee replacement (TKR), it's a different matter. The surgical approach to the joint is more extensive, involving the quadriceps muscle in a major way. It produces more pain, certainly for the first weeks after surgery. Isotonic exercises may involve stretching out tissues, and even early adhesions. This generally is painful. But the degree of pain should lessen dramatically over this period.

With THR and Resurf surgery, the pain is usually not deep seated, but instead relates to the surgical incision. With TKRs and knee Resurfs, the pain tends to be more profound, involving the body of the quadriceps.

In either case, if serious pain goes on for more than the first week or so of exercise/rehabilitation, it is time to see your surgeon.

Ancillary and Critical Insider General Tips

In the first days of exercise, I don't like my patients to "ice down" after exercise. (See "The Old R.I.C.E. Formula" on page 118.)

Instead, I suggest they observe the amount of swelling and/or heat, and particularly take note of the nature of any pain or aching. If persistent or severe, it is a warning to be both respected and reported. It will shortly subside on its own, particularly if you rest and elevate the extremity for a short while. Above all do not dream of using compression, such as by the use of an elasticized knee brace.

Also, do not start any exercise with weight resistance, no matter how light. Even if you've been able to work with weights prior to surgery, post surgery you'll need to drop back to the increasing reps mode, before adding weight.

Pay attention to your dressing, especially after an exercise session. If you are going to drain fluid, it will be after your

The Old R.I.C.E Formula

Those of you who've suffered athletic-type injuries, undoubtedly know this formula. It is the golden treatment touted by many coaches and therapists. Spelled out, it consists of:

R for rest

I for icing

C for compression

E for elevation

However, in the recovery period from a total or partial joint replacement, only the "R" and "E" are useful. As an orthopedist I have never wanted my post-op patients to use either ice or compression.

Ice is really only useful in an immediate injury to a joint, muscle, or tendon or in an inflammatory condition. Using ice other than as a very mild analgesia lies in the realm of myth, despite its widespread practice.

After exercise, or even just at the end of the day after standing or sitting, *elevation* and *rest* are not only comforting, but can also help reduce any swelling the day may have brought.

"reps." Take note of color and amount and report to your surgeon. Normally there should be slight to none.

During post-exercise bathing (showering), you must find a way to "waterproof" your dressing, or "French bathe" (top to bottom with wash cloth or sponge at basin). Ask your surgeon (he's your wound master) how long you'll need to wait before the surgical closure can be exposed to water. And, of course, always dry carefully after aqueous exposure.

If, for whatever reason, you've not been able to do pre-op exercise, or if you've been very limited due to arthritis or any other medical condition, you may expect some soreness after exercises. It should measure mild on the Richter scale and may respond to warm (not hot), wet heat.

About Walkers and Crutches

Be sure your walker or crutches are correctly adjusted for your height. This is best done by a physical therapist, but a surgical supply person also knows how to do it.

Personally, I find Canadian or Lofstrand forearm crutches much easier to use than conventional under-arm ones. Even when they're padded, conventional crutches can produce sore armpits. As to fit, the cuff should come to about 1 inch below the elbow or 2 inches above.

About Canes

These are balancing/stabilizing, not weight-supporting, devices. They also serve to let the general public know that you're a recovering walker.

Again, be sure it's the right height for you. The top bend of the cane should be at the level of the crease of your wrist when you have your arm relaxed by the side of your body. A rubber tip is all important. A cane is usually used opposite your operated leg.

About Chairs

If you have had a THR, you will want a raised seat, or at least not a low chair. The reason is that too much flexion for the first few months after surgery can actually lead to a hip dislocation.

Obviously you want a very sturdy chair, and one that doesn't slip along the floor. Some padding, if it's thin and attached, makes for comfort. Loose pillowing can be treacherous, giving way when least expected.

I like a straight wooden chair with arms. The arms can be used for upper extremity exercise.

Setting Your Posthab Goals

I know it may to be tempting, particularly for THRs and hip Resurf patients, to set early high rehab standards. After all, the fact that your once very painful and limited joint is now working is a treat. *But,* let your muscles and endurance come on slowly and steadily. Again, it's a matter of recognizing that in order to fix the affected joint your surgeon had to cut into and through muscles, capsules, and other soft-tissue structures. Give them the chance to come back into their own at a reasonable pace. The ancient Romans had it perfectly: *Festina Lente,* which means the race will go to the tortoise, not the hare.

Your rate of progress is individual. There is no solid gold standard of time or accomplishment when it comes to post-op recovery.

Considerations relevant to your progress are:

• Pre-op condition and conditioning practices.
• Age (believe me, 80-year-olds take more time and patience than 50-year-olds).
• Other medical conditions (such as cardiac or respiratory limitations).
• Surgical complication of the procedure.
• There must be others—I leave it to you.

Posthab Exercises

After any surgery, life is altered for a while. Your body has to have time to recover from even minor surgeries, because even the minor ones are perceived by the body as an invasion and it

Absolute No-No's for Posthabbers

1. Never cross your legs or adduct them to more than neutral.
2. Do not flex you hips more than 90 degrees.
3. Do nothing that "jogs" your hip repeatedly (Running, contact sports, football, tennis, moguls, etc.)

reacts accordingly. *Hip replacement surgery recovery* can be especially intense.

Temporary changes in bodily function may include a poor appetite. It's important to consume plenty of liquids (water, juice, milk, and light soups) to prevent dehydration. Don't worry, you'll want solid food again soon enough.

You might experience some insomnia as well. This is normal. Try not to take too many naps during the day so that you'll be sufficiently sleepy at night.

Pain medicine contains narcotics, which can cause constipation. Eating lots of fruit, particularly prunes, can help. Use stool softeners or laxatives such as milk of magnesia only as a last resort.

Ways of controlling the normal discomfort that occurs after hip replacement surgery include taking your pain medicine at least half an hour prior to your physical therapy sessions and gradually weaning yourself from your prescription medication to an over-the-counter drug such as Tylenol. Two extra-strength Tylenol for example, can be substituted for the prescription drug up to four times a day.

Physical therapy will begin a day or two after your surgery. Part of rehabilitation includes Occupational Therapy. O.T. includes Activities of Daily Living (ADLs) such as getting in to and out of bed, bathing, and getting dressed.

You will probably need special equipment in order to achieve total independence. This equipment includes adaptive bathing and dressing aids. Other common ADL tools are reachers, sock aids, long shoe horns, long sponges, and elastic shoelaces. You can obtain these items prior to surgery; they can be found at most medical supply stores.

As your physical therapy becomes less supervised, your home exercise program will become even more essential to you. Your goals for that first four to six weeks after surgery include:

Ankle Rotations (Ankle Circles)

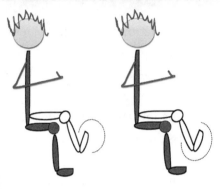

Sitting in a chair:

- Move your ankle inward toward your other foot and then outward away from your other foot. (Clockwise and then Counter clockwise)
- Do not rotate your knee—just your ankle.
- Repeat 5 times in each direction.

Bed-Supported Knee Bends

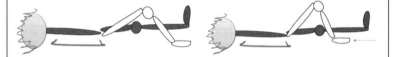

Lying in bed:

- Slide your heel toward your buttocks, bending your knee and keeping your heel on the bed. (For some patients be cautious of rubbing your heel too hard as this may cause unwanted friction.)
- Do not let your knee roll inward nor let your hip exceed 90 degrees.
- Repeat this exercise 10 times

Buttock Contractions (Butt Squeeze Lying Down

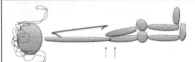

Lying in bed:

- Tighten buttock muscles and hold to a count of 5.
- Simply tighten you butt muscles (a sort of clench), if performing correctly you will feel yourself "rise" slightly in the bed
- Repeat this exercise 10 times.

Hip Abduction Exercise

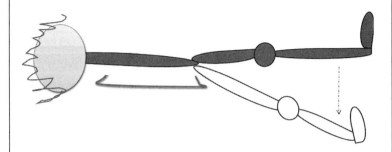

Lying in bed:

* Slide your operated leg out to the side as far as you can and then back.
* Repeat this exercise 10 times.

Standing Knee Raises

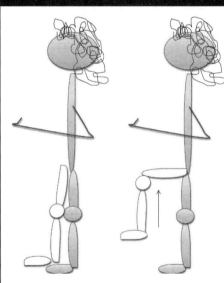

This one you have to stand for – so let's stand up.

Find anything sturdy that can serve as a support, but leaving your lower body free. Ideally, something like the back of a sturdy chair, kitchen table, or anything that can serve as the barre used by ballet dancers to support yourself.

* Lift your operated leg toward your chest.
* Do not lift your knee higher than your waist.
* Hold for a count of 2 or 3 and put your leg down.

Standing Hip Extensions

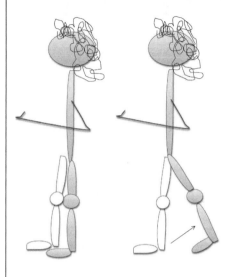

Again, find anything sturdy that can serve as a support, but leaving your lower body free.

- Lift your operated leg backward slowly.
- Try to keep your back straight.
- Hold for a count of 2 or 3 and then return your foot to the floor

Standing Hip Abduction

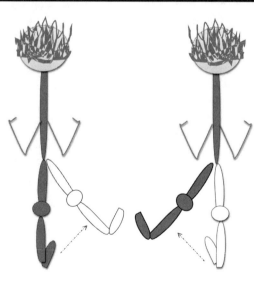

Again, find anything sturdy that can serve as a support, leaving your lower body free – like a chair back.

- Be sure your hip, knee, and foot are pointing straight forward.

- Keep your body straight. With your knee straight, lift your operated leg out to the side.
- Slowly lower your leg so your foot is back on the floor.

Sitting in a chair:
- Bend ankles up toward your body as far as possible
- Now point toe away from your body. (Step on gas pedal)

Chapter Twelve Highlights

- Check out needed equipment with O.T.
- Check out continuing P.T. wherever it is arranged.
- Check out visiting nurse service and home making if needed.

Your Space

_____

_____

_____

_____

_____

_____

_____

_____

The First Few Months

It usually takes a few months before you re-accept yourself as a person again, rather than a patient. The key to getting there is to *be patient, and don't take chances.* Think ahead before you do anything new or different. This may sound like advice from an over-protective mother hen, but I assure you it's not. You really can dislocate your hip by ignoring your hip cautions, particularly during the first six months after surgery.

You will still be on crutches or using a walker, and this will continue for anywhere from 6 to 12 weeks. Stairs, especially more than 8 to 10 steps at a pop, will be slow, awkward, and may be taxing.

You will tire easily, and probably nap in the afternoon, as your endurance will be limited. It might be best if you limit day-to-day ambitions to allow for your current limitations. Nevertheless, walk every day and try to increase your distance a little every day; for city dwellers, this means adding about a half block more per walk.

Your sleep habits may take a while to re-establish. I used a mild sleeping medication, Ambien. Some of my patients liked melatonin, Benadryl, or Lunesta, and there are others. Don't hesitate to take something to help you sleep; a good rest at night is a pearl beyond price in this phase of your recovery.

Remember, you must sleep with a pillow between your legs for a minimum of 12 weeks—and on your back if possible!

Use Caution and Accept Help with Your Daily Activities

You will be more dependent on help than you might have thought, especially home-making help. Don't fuss. Thank whoever comes to your aid and accept it. Your first few days, use a dressing, bathing, walking buddy. Showers or sponge baths are okay, but no tub. Remember to use rubber mats in the bathroom and shower. Have your loose clothing close at hand.

You will need to think about how to do some things that have been automatic in the past.

Oddly enough, home is a place of some hazard, simply because most of us take for granted that we can automatically function and get around in it. The familiar can become full of risk for this reason. It's ironic, since we always think of home as a shelter, not a challenge.

You really *must* think about everything you do for the first few weeks and how you do it, and consider whether or not it poses a risk.

- Is the bottom shelf too low when you want something from it, and your grabber is in the other room?
- Do you have to twist to get quickly from the stove to the sink?
- Is the step ladder well balanced or rickety?
- Did I remember to put my cell phone by my side?

I leave you to fill in the rest of the blanks. I'm not familiar with your home; only you know your layout and daily routines and what may present a hazard.

No matter how slick you are on crutches, assume that you're a klutz for the first weeks at home, and make allowances for it. You may also feel tired and lazy, so be sure the telephone, your crutches, and your grabber are all always within your reach.

You'll also need to hold off on travel, demanding professional projects, and full-activity commitments for a minimum of one or two months after surgery. And be sure to try walking without crutches at home before even thinking about trying it elsewhere.

About Sex

Over the years of treating THR patients, there were always two invariable questions: the first was, "Will I die on the operating table?" and the second, "When will I be able to have sex?" The answer to the first was no; the answer to the second was—yes, by all means, as soon as you have the energy.

But in the small-caution department, don't hang from the chandelier, and do use the missionary position. Lying on your back with your legs akimbo, whether male or female, puts you at no risk, at least from dislocation, and presuming all the other usual precautions have been observed. Other approaches, such as manual or oral sex, are also safe as toast.

For those of you who are "Kama Sutra" hip, the following positions are iffy for the first few weeks: Indrani, Milk and Water, The Lotus, Suspended Congress, Splitting of a Bamboo, and a Pair of Tongs. Another chancy position to be avoided for the first six months or so is the doggy position, as you may over-flex your hips on this one. But on the six-month anniversary of your surgery, you may give it all a go!

Your List of *Don'ts*

You've heard it before, but let's review. *Don't:*

- Flex or bend beyond 90 degrees.
- Cross your legs.
- Ignore pain when you move or do something.
- Ignore the slightest fever.
- Internally rotate at your hips (in-turn).

Your List of *Dos*

You've heard these as well, but here we go:

- Check your doctor and P.T. schedules. Professional and domestic demands will have to be made around these for the first month or two. Consider posting these in an obvious spot and on your calendar.
- Remember, your first surgical visit will be within two to three weeks. You'll be x-rayed and, if staples or sutures have not been previously removed, they'll be taken out.
- When you get ready to go back to work, modify transportation as needed to accommodate crutches and prevent hyper-flexion. Remember the protective techniques you were taught for getting in and out of cars and cabs.
- Speaking of weather, when it snows or sleets or even rains, have your meals home-delivered from your favorite restaurant. Do anything other than schlep around in bad weather for the first few months, at least during the time you're crutch- or cane-dependent.

Don't schedule invasive procedures for the first four to six months after surgery unless you absolutely have to. If a minor infection were to set up, even if distant from your hip, it could nevertheless seed infection directly to your prosthesis. Remember that your prosthesis, although made of inert material, is still a foreign body that may serve as a subject of infection. Dentistry (even a thorough cleaning), a gynecological or proctologic examination, and cosmetic procedures are to be considered invasive after a THR and must be covered with antibiotics 24 hours before and 24 hours after being done.

Traveling after Hip Surgery

Travel can be burdensome during the time you are still on crutches. Handling luggage, waiting in line, and hailing a cab all become unduly difficult. If you *must* travel, follow this advice when possible.

By Air

Travel by air has become a matter of misery, quantities of your time misspent and egregious delays in overcrowded airports. So what more can we add to your enjoyment? Seriously, though, you need to think your travel by air through.

- *Order a wheelchair!* When you book your ticket, tell the airline that you'll need a wheelchair on both ends of your flight. Check any luggage you might ordinarily carry on. Travel for a recent THR recipient is slow at best, so the delay to retrieve your bags fits right in.
- Book an aisle seat, if possible in the first row in the section, so you're bothered as little as possible by other passengers moving about.
- Plan for extra time in the airport to have the airline get a wheelchair to you and wheel you through luggage check or passport control or whatever. If you usually schedule two hours before flight time at the airport, add another hour to this time.
- On a long flight, go through some of your "in-bed" exercises, for your calves and buttocks, and do some marching in place right in your seat.
- Schedule trips to the bathroom at times of little use (e.g., during the film, or, for long flights, late at night or early in the morning).

By Train or Bus

Wheelchairs are not easily used in these situations. But if you've graduated to a cane for walking, revert back to crutches for purposes of the trip. Using crutches will tend to keep people at more of a distance, and you may have to do more walking and standing than you're used to. With respect to the giant step, you may have to climb to get into a bus or train car, as kneeling buses only descend so far.

- Ask another passenger or car attendant to take your luggage aboard. If traveling by train, a trainman will stow it for you.
- Get another kind soul to literally give you a gentle boost (not a shove), once you've got your best foot and leg up on the step. I think people still like helping when they can see their help makes a material and immediate difference.
- Try for a seat close to the door of the train car.
- When getting off the train, reverse the same process as boarding.

Even if you don't normally use a porter for trains, if you can get one, it's the way to go. Or have a friend or family member go with you to the station on departure and meet you on arrival. If this is not possible when traveling by bus, perhaps a fellow passenger can help with luggage through the station.

Much of what I've suggested in this chapter is simple common sense that you may have already thought of, but it is extremely important.

At the end of three to four months, you'll be crutch-free, walking a quarter of a mile without trouble, able to climb most stairs, use public transportation, shop as you like, and even begin to resume easy sports activities.

Hopefully you'll be doing some consistent exercise program at least four times per week and preferably daily. Regular exercise, particularly range-of-motion exercise—is important to the proper maintenance of your new hip. The operated muscles about the hip and the capsule of the hip will have a tendency to stiffen without exercise. As you already know, I strongly suggest swimming when you can, and riding a stationary bicycle with resistance set low and timer set long.

For me, high-impact sports are a permanent no-no. The risk of dislocation of the THR or fracture on the same side is too much and always too present to warrant the action. Non-contact, low-impact sports, such as cross-country skiing, are fine. In the problematic group, and for my patients, I strongly discourage sports and such games as squash or paddle ball (too much sudden stopping and starting), mountain climbing (especially with rappelling), most team sports, weight-lifting, and extensive, marathon-type running.

Personally, I am against jogging or running after THR. It isn't that you can't get by with them; you can. But it's not really smart to pound on the mechanism you have taken great pains to install. Jogging and distance running challenge your THR or Resurf, especially if done frequently and for long periods. If there is no reasonable access to a heated pool, there is another terrific exercise alternative—fast walking.

I strongly advise against contact sports, including but not limited to basketball, lacrosse, hockey, boxing, wrestling, judo, Tai chi, and so-called touch football. Have I forgotten something? I think you can evaluate other sports, given the above list as an indication.

Horseback riding is another very questionable activity. Doubles tennis and handball are okay. If you're willing to take chances, downhill skiing is a possibility, but never ski competitively, and preferably stick to just the gentlest runs (typically labeled as greens and blues). Get a scooper/retriever for golf balls in the cup—it won't count as a 15th club. Remember, do nothing that involves a full squat.

There are always new sports to try. Perhaps you never gave golf a shot. I want to tell you it's a fascinating sport. Jack

Nicklaus and Arnie Palmer both have THRs. Before starting any new athletic activities for the first year, it's a good idea to check it out with your surgeon.

You'll have seen your surgeon for at least two check-ups and an x-ray by now. Be sure to ask any leftover questions. I liked to see and examine my patients at three weeks, six weeks, three months, and 1 year. I took x-rays with each visit. I loved it when a patient scheduled a 3-year or 6-year visit. And I don't think I'm alone in liking this re-visit schedule.

Above all, if you pick up on any minor glitches, twinges, limitations, or problems, call your surgeon and get them checked out. If you'd bought a new car, you would be discussing minor gremlins with your car dealer, so, in the same spirit, check out your THR with the surgeon who installed it.

Having said that, as good as we've gotten with both THRs or Resurfs, only God makes a perfect hip.

Chapter Thirteen Highlights

- Don't get impatient, and do remember to sleep with an adduction pillow.
- Use travel precautions in planes, trains, and automobiles.
- Sex—by all means, but check cautions given in this chapter.

Your Space

_____

_____

_____

_____

_____

_____

_____

_____

_____

_____

_____

_____

_____

_____

_____

_____

THR and Resurf Odds and Ends

This chapter contains some thoughts that don't seem to fit neatly under any other heading but are still issues and questions that may come up for you in the months and years after your hip replacement.

Metal Detectors

A question almost all patients ask is: "Will my THR set off the metal detector in the airport?" The answer is usually no, but it depends on the scanner's sensitivity. Mine never has, and I have traveled extensively in the United States and abroad. The Orient I cannot answer for, but if worse comes to worst, you can always flash your THR scar (just kidding!) or simply carry a letter or ID-type card from your surgeon. Although certainly part of your hip is a metal alloy, the layers of soft tissue over it may prevent the detector from going off.

Ectopic Calcification

There's a post-op phenomenon called "ectopic calcification," which is when extra bone develops around your THR following surgery. It's not been established exactly why this happens. Thankfully, it's highly unusual, but when it occurs and is left untended, it can freeze up your hip with an irregular bony formation. Again, this is a rare occurrence, but if you have any history of this kind of calcific formation around previous fracture sites, it's logical that you may be at some risk.

Your surgeon may want to consider early post-op irradiation or preventative treatment within the first week or so after surgery. Otherwise, since your surgeon schedules regular post-op x-rays, this calcification should be detected in its early stages. The jury is out on treatment, and the ideas are in constant change, but irradiation and chemical anti-growth medications are among the therapies. The percentage of occurrence is way below .01 percent, and that's why it's included here under "odds and ends"—really as an observation rather than a caution.

Robotic Implantation of THR

There has been discussion in medical and non-medical literature of the use of partial robotic implantation of a THR. I have reservations about this idea. It sounds very technologically advanced, but . . . in essence, every patient and every THR is highly individual and requires individual surgical technique, selections, and device insertion.

Currently we're simply not that advanced in the human/computer physical interface, but who knows what the future will provide in this area. For myself, I think there is nothing quite like the attention and experience of an individual surgeon. I'm not sure that this factor is replaceable by the mathematical model, even with sophisticated variables. So, at the moment I see no reason to get excited about the robot surgeon as a technical breakthrough. I can see where it might be helpful with the mini-hips, but I've already expressed how I feel about these.

My suggestion in the area of THRs is to look for a better cat, not a better mousetrap, to coin a phrase. There is nothing like an experienced THR or Resurf surgeon with a good track record to get the job done.

Speaking of the foreseeable future, there is no solution other than a THR for a distorted and arthritic hip joint—no magic natural joint restorer, and no magical medication to take care of the problem today.

THR Revision

THR revisions, or "re-dos" as surgeons sometimes refer to them, are a very different kettle of fish from the initial THR procedure. Here are the most common causes.

Dislocations within the First Few Days to Months

These can occur very early or later within the first few months and are often caused by an inadvertent in-turning or over-flexion. The hip can usually be put back into place (reduction) under sedation, followed by use of an abduction splint (one step up from pillows between the legs) for two to three months. Most surgeons will treat a repeat of such a dislocation in the same way, with reduction under general anesthesia and, again, an abduction splint. However, after the third dislocation, a re-do THR is performed, often with a different type of socket. This usually does the trick.

Infection

A still sorrier and even more complex problem is infection, which can and often does result in the need for replacement of the prosthetic hip joint. After the infected hip has been opened, the surgeon must remove the THR device and debride the infected tissue. The joint must be drained, and the bacteria cultured and identified so that the infection can be treated with the appropriate antibiotic. Currently there is no absolutely agreed-upon timing for when a new hip can be placed after the infection has been treated.

The surgeon must be sure there are no lingering traces of the bug that caused the infection before he or she replaces the hip. Often this is established by repeat cultures of the wound drainage, sometimes followed with another open clean-out procedure at the time or a few days before the placement of the new THR.

There are surgeons who try to avoid removing the prosthesis by treating the infection with massive doses of antibiotics alone, or with a combination of these antibiotics and a limited incision and drainage, and a second set of cultures. Sometimes this works. If it does, it means that all or part of the original THR may be retained. However, this is not the accepted protocol by all surgeons at this time.

INSIDER TIP

The Matter of Re-Do Surgeons

If you've been reluctant to do an in-depth research into your surgeon's background and credentials before having a THR or Resurf, for a re-do it's a necessity!

You must determine a surgeon's re-do record in no uncertain terms. A novice may get by with a first go, but never a re-do. A re-do is not a simple replacement of one prosthesis for another. It is a far more complicated surgical problem to try to solve.

Whatever problems existed during your first surgery, the chances of problems are more than doubled with a re-do.

In general, it may not be the wisest choice to go back to the same surgeon who did your initial procedure. Often a fresh look and approach may serve you better.

The *optimal treatment* for an infected THR has yet to be established; there is no unanimity on the treatment protocol. But, whichever treatment path your doctor selects, in all likelihood you may be faced with a second THR placement.

Wear and Tear

Another scenario that may call for a revision is the aging of the THR components, which can result in them loosening or wearing out. You may hear the term *aseptic necrosis*; this means that the bone surrounding the prosthetic component is dying, which can be seen on x-ray. Additionally, the degraded material from the socket may get in between the device and the surrounding bone, causing loosening, or occasionally the stem of the prosthesis cracks or breaks. In cemented THRs, the cement mantle may fail. When any of these things occur, you will need a THR revision or "re-do."

I wish I could say that the second round is as easy and relatively complication-free as the first. But it just isn't so.

- The rate of infection is two to three times what it is for a first hip.
- The life expectancy of a re-do is half that of a first.
- The range of motion of a re-do is less than that of a first.

There are soft-tissue disadvantages to a second surgery in the same area, such as additional scar tissue formation, deep as well as superficial. This may contribute to lack of power to the muscles involved as well as lost flexibility and diminished range of motion.

Operative blood loss is generally more than in the first surgery, because operating through scar tissue produces more bleeding than operating on normal muscle and subcutaneous tissue.

Other surgical risks (e.g., pulmonary embolism, allergic reactions, and so on) are generally the same. The satisfaction rating falls from the high 90 percents for a first-time THR to around 60 to 70 percent for a second one, at best.

So, now that I've given you the bad news about revision THRs, maybe a little ray of light would be welcome. As the population ages, there will be an increased demand for THRs. Therefore, the number of surgeons and their THR skill pool will increase to meet this demand. It's the capitalistic, American way of doing things. Also, companies that design and manufacture THR implants are always seeking to be on the cutting edge (excuse the pun) of technology.

The surgical approach of Dr. John Charnley, inventor of the modern THR, has basically not altered much in 40-some-odd years, but the implants have been improved markedly in strength, adaptability, and durability—and they continue to do so!

As the number of THRs increases, so does the number of re-dos. Clinical research is looking into ways to address the problems raised by re-dos, even as we speak. Surgeons are a proud, and sometimes vain, lot (one may quibble, but sometimes this vanity works to the patient's advantage) who wish to avoid "poor" and "mediocre" results in their records. They are perpetually driven to seek better surgical and technical solutions to their problems. In time, surgeons will likely solve the difficulties associated with revision hip surgery with their "smarts" and scalpels.

To finish on a lighter note, recently I went to dinner with two friends who had also had THRs, and one of them a revision THR. As often happens, we were discussing details of current activity, x-rays, and all the usual talk among THR "alumni." The friend with the revision THR was several months beyond what had to be considered a very successful result, and he called for after-dinner cognac all around. When the drinks arrived, he proposed the toast, "Here's to successful THRs and many more!" To which I could only reply, as I hope you will, "Hip, hip, hooray!"

Chapter Fourteen Highlights

- Dislocations may occur anytime from the first few days to the first few months—check precautions against.
- Revisions may be occasioned by repeated dislocations, infection, or other difficulties—revisions are never as good as the first time around.
- Check out ASAP any post-op squeaking, clunking, clicking, and other odd sounds from your hip.

Your Space

_____

_____

_____

_____

_____

_____

_____

_____

_____

_____

_____

Chapter Fifteen

The Future Hip...
An Educated Guess

In the last 20 years, the progress in THRs and Resurfs has been a matter of better devices made of more enduring, better-tolerated, and better-functioning materials.

Surgeons and manufacturers are constantly testing and trying to improve implants. And surgeons are always trying to simplify the procedure, as well as make it safer for patients and shorten recovery time. I can say with a certain amount of pride that to a large extent they have succeeded in these goals, to the benefit of patients.

I think the future, however, will focus on the most common problem that necessitates hip surgery: osteoarthritis. If we become able to restore the cartilage of the hip joint and the quality of the bone, replacement surgery might be obviated; if not permanently, then for a significant period of time.

So, stem-cell research enters. The stem cell, no matter its source, is an omnipotent generalized cell that usually goes on to develop into a specialized cell. In other words, a stem cell is the universal precursor cell that can become muscle, bone, cartilage, or any other type of human cell. It follows then that if we can reliably re-grow or restore the hip's cartilage, we restore its ability to move and glide, and hence reverse the end effect of arthritis.

Having suggested a true cartilage repair or restoration, we could then take cells from, say, the mouth, and culture and grow them to become an entire cartilage tissue ready to be used in a decimated hip. A technique, in effect, could then be used to emplace or inject these stem cells directly into the cartilage of the hip joint, recreating the normal structure.

Obviously, this last suggestion may not be a possibility now. But as of this writing, platelet-rich plasma is being harvested from blood and given back to patients in a purified and concentrated form. It is not yet FDA-approved for humans, although some pro footballers have tried it in order to hasten ligament and tendon repair. It has also been tried on horses with reported good results. Perhaps, in time, it could be used for the soft tissues of the hip or knee.

But, who ever dreamed that mold on a piece of stale bread could produce penicillin? It's one of the world's most effective antibiotics, which now cures diseases and infections from which people once routinely died!

Pediatricians almost invariably examine newborn hips for hip dyscrasias, which may be present even at birth. In the future, such children might be monitored for early treatment or intervention before arthritis becomes full blown. Much research is also being done on in-utero gene therapy. I have wandered astray from your hips to those of your grandchildren, for which I must apologize, but the horizon is never as far away as one thinks.

Knowledge in medicine is the one growing constant. In our climb to knowledge, we stand upon the shoulders of those who have gone before us. And so we remember them and return to thank all of these imaginative and caring physicians. For without them we might still be seeking the solutions they researched and found for so many illnesses.

As both patient and practitioner, I wish to be the first in line to thank them. May the future be bright.

Chapter Sixteen

Your Hip Surgery Organizer

Initial Consultation with Your Surgeon

Your initial consultation is your first chance to get to know your surgeon and his or her staff and learn about what they can do for you. Your first visit will be very in-depth, and you should plan to stay for at least 45 minutes or so, depending on the complexity of your problem.

During this initial visit, your surgeon and staff will take a comprehensive medical history. This visit gives you the opportunity to obtain your surgeon's opinions on the type of surgery you require, responses to your questions, and explanation of the risks associated with your procedure.

Please Bring the Following Items:

❑ Family members/friends/significant others whom you would like to be present as "second ears" and prompters to aid on your behalf.

❑ A detailed list of your current medications.

❑ Any x-rays or studies taken of your hip by previous physicians that can be acquired.

❑ List of physicians you have visited in the past three years with all contact information.

❑ A *written* list of the questions you have for your surgeon.

Current Medicine List

Medicine _____	Medicine _____
Dose _____	Dose _____
Times Taken _____	Times Taken _____
Allergy_____	Allergy _____
Reaction _____	Reaction _____
Medicine _____	Medicine _____
Dose _____	Dose _____
Times Taken _____	Times Taken _____
Allergy_____	Allergy _____
Reaction _____	Reaction _____
Medicine _____	Medicine _____
Dose _____	Dose _____
Times Taken _____	Times Taken _____
Allergy_____	Allergy _____
Reaction _____	Reaction _____
Medicine _____	Medicine _____
Dose _____	Dose _____
Times Taken _____	Times Taken _____
Allergy_____	Allergy _____
Reaction _____	Reaction _____

Prehab Exercise Log

If you are preparing for a new hip you should talk to your doctor or physical therapist about creating an exercise program best-fit for you as an individual. Despite what you may feel about independence and self-help, let a physical therapist show you what will work and how to execute even simple exercises. It is your guarantee you will do nothing to cause more harm, and that what you are doing is entirely within your competence.

Your Prehab program will include strengthening your arms and shoulders, which will help you cope with crutches or a walker after surgery. Others will help maintain the strength of your leg muscles. The exercises should take about 20 minutes to complete, and if possible, you should do them twice a day.

Quadriceps Sitting Kicks (page 66)

Reps	Mon.	Tue.	Wed.	Thu.	Fri.	Sat.	Sun.
Week 1							
Week 2							
Week 3							
Week 4							

Quadriceps Isotonic Sitting Kicks with Weights (page 66)

Reps	Mon.	Tue.	Wed.	Thu.	Fri.	Sat.	Sun.
Week 1							
Week 2							
Week 3							
Week 4							

Gastrocs Isotonic Calf Press (page 67)

Reps	Mon.	Tue.	Wed.	Thu.	Fri.	Sat.	Sun.
Week 1							
Week 2							
Week 3							
Week 4							

Gastrocs Isotonic Calf Press with Weights (page 67)

Reps	Mon.	Tue.	Wed.	Thu.	Fri.	Sat.	Sun.
Week 1							
Week 2							
Week 3							
Week 4							

Gluteus Maximus Squeeze (page 68)

Reps	Mon.	Tue.	Wed.	Thu.	Fri.	Sat.	Sun.
Week 1							
Week 2							
Week 3							
Week 4							

Abductor Sets (page 68)

Reps	Mon.	Tue.	Wed.	Thu.	Fri.	Sat.	Sun.
Week 1							
Week 2							
Week 3							
Week 4							

Abdominal Squeeze (page 69)

Reps	Mon.	Tue.	Wed.	Thu.	Fri.	Sat.	Sun.
Week 1							
Week 2							
Week 3							
Week 4							

Chair Pushups (page 69)

Reps	Mon.	Tue.	Wed.	Thu.	Fri.	Sat.	Sun.
Week 1							
Week 2							
Week 3							
Week 4							

Questions to Ask Your Surgeon

1. What is the operation (procedure) that is recommended?

   _____

   _____

2. What is the surgeon's experience with this type of operation?_____

   _____

3. Are there alternatives to surgery? _____

   _____

4. What type of anesthesia is required for the procedure?

   _____

   _____

5. What are the specific risks and benefits of this procedure?

   _____

   _____

6. What about a second opinion? And where can I get one?

   _____

   _____

7. What is the recovery process after this procedure? _____

   _____

   _____

8. Where will the operation be done? _____

   _____

   _____

9. Is this procedure covered by my insurance plan?_____

   _____

   _____

10. How much will the operation cost? _____

   _____

   _____

Important Names & Numbers

Surgeon _____
      Phone _____ Email _____
      Address _____

Internist _____
      Phone _____ Email _____
      Address _____

Hospital _____
      Phone _____ Email _____
      Address _____

Admitting Office _____
      Phone _____ Email _____
      Address _____

Nursing Station _____
      Phone _____ Email _____
      Address _____

Nursing Office _____
      Phone _____ Email _____
      Address _____

Hospital Floor Head Nurse _____

    Phone _____ Email _____

    Address _____

Physical Therapist _____

    Phone _____ Email _____

    Address _____

Occupational Therapist _____

    Phone _____ Email _____

    Address _____

Rental Supply Store _____

    Phone _____ Email _____

    Address _____

Home Physical Therapist _____

    Phone _____ Email _____

    Address _____

Home Aide _____

    Phone _____ Email _____

    Address _____

Insurance Contact _____

    Phone _____ Email _____

    Address _____

Hip-Proof Your House Checklist

House

❑ Remove all loose rugs.

❑ Make clear pathways from bed to front door, bathroom to kitchen, etc.

❑ Raise your bed on blocks or arrange for a hospital bed to be delivered.

❑ Raise your favorite chair somewhere near the TV, or arrange to rent these items.

❑ Put a table in the hall for newspaper/mail; you don't want to stoop or squat to get them.

❑ Install handrails in the shower and near the toilet.

❑ Put non-slip mats in the shower or bath tub.

❑ Have a cell phone or hands-free phone ready for use.

❑ Place all pots and pans, dishwashing supplies, etc., at waist height—the lower shelves in your kitchen, oven, and refrigerator are all forbidden territory.

❑ Clean house as thoroughly as possible.

Housekeeping

❑ Be sure medications are near the sink, easy to reach; have at least a 3-week supply on hand.

❑ Stock up on lots of frozen food.

❑ Arrange clothes, cardigan sweaters, loafers, or slip-on shoes where you can get them easily.

❑ Make sure you have at least 1 week's worth of pet food. Also arrange your pet's food and water dish above floor level. Normal pet-care responsibilities must be given to a friend, partner, dog walker, or whomever—not you—for at least 6 weeks.

❑ Stop newspaper delivery during your hospitalization, or have a friend pick them up along with the mail.

❑ Arrange banking so that you (or your partner) have access to cash for 3 weeks after your release from the hospital.

❑ Get a backpack for toting things around; this frees your hands.

Pre Surgery Checklist

6 to 8 Weeks Prior to Surgery

❑ Arrange for a morning surgery time. Ask your surgeon to book a time slot as early in the day as possible on the surgical schedule.

❑ Start arranging your absence from work. Inform all who must know, and to help arrange your coverage.

❑ Arrange for car driving. Since you will be unable to drive following your surgery, you should make advance transportation arrangements for 8 to 10 weeks.

❑ Have minor surgical and dental procedures done. Make time to get to the dentist for any necessary cleaning, caps, or any oral surgery or procedure.

❑ Arrange for house and pet sitting. Count on being in the hospital for 5 to 6 days, but it will be another 6 weeks until you're able to feed and water things, and at least 2 to 3 months before you're ready to walk your dog.

❑ Make an appointment to pre-donate your blood. You won't actually pre-donate until about three to four weeks before surgery, but now is when you should find out exactly where to go, the hours, and the procedures required to do so.

2 to 3 Weeks Prior to Surgery

❑ Complete the blood donation.

❑ Check on your private nursing arrangement, if you've made one.

❑ Talk to the admitting office about your accommodation; state your preference regarding two-bed, four-bed, private room, or open ward.

❑ Finalize home and work arrangements.

❑ Change blood thinners (if you're taking them) 1 to 2 weeks before surgery, exactly as your internist has directed.

❑ Stop taking anti-inflammatory medication at least 2 weeks prior to surgery. You can switch to a medication that won't interfere with your blood clotting or coagulation (e.g., Tylenol). If you fail to do this, you could end up losing a great deal more blood on the operating table than you need. This is a risk you don't want to chance, even having reserved some of your own blood.

❑ Report immediately to your surgeon any infections, either general or local (anything from a urinary tract infection or gall bladder attack to a boil, rash, or skin breakdown).

❑ Report immediately to your surgeon any change in your general medical status.

❑ Talk to both your anesthesiologist and internist about your long-term medical regimen and what to do about it for the last few weeks before surgery, and especially the day of surgery.

One Week Prior to Hospital Admission

❑ Organize personal care items such as toothbrush, tooth-paste, denture cleanser, comb, skin-care products, deodor-ant, make-up, shaving kit, personal toiletries.

❑ Locate flat, supportive athletic, or walking shoes that are non-slip.

❑ Pack nightwear such as a short nightgown, robe, loose pajamas, baggy shorts.

❑ Be sure you have clothing that fits over dressings such as socks, undergarments, shirts, pants, sweatshirts, cardigan-type sweaters.

❑ Plan to wear eyeglasses instead of contact lenses, as they are easier to take off and less likely to be lost. If you plan to wear contacts, bring storage containers and all necessary products.

❑ Hospital rooms usually have TV and phone, but you may want to bring two of the same book/magazine (just in case one gets lost).

❑ Don't bring valuables; leave them at home. When it comes to money, you may want to bring only a small amount for newspapers and a blank check or credit card for buying any medical care equipment.

❑ Some hospitals provide a container for dentures; if not, bring your own. Keep the container in a drawer or bedside table, not on the bed or food tray.

❑ Organize clothing you plan to wear home, including shoes, socks, undergarments, loose shirts, and sweat pants.

❑ Be sure to pack this book!

Hip Surgery Calendar

Date	Event	Comments
_____	Blood Donation	_____
		_____
_____	Day of Admission	_____
		_____
_____	Day of Surgery	_____
		_____
_____	Went Home	_____
		_____
_____	First Quarter Mile (3 blocks)	_____
		_____
_____	First Car Drive	_____
		_____
_____	No Extra Home Help	_____
		_____
_____	First Trip	_____
		_____
_____	1st Post-Op Appointment	_____
		_____
_____	2nd Post-Op Appointment	_____
		_____
_____	3rd Post-Op Appointment	_____
		_____
_____	No Crutches	_____
		_____
_____	No Cane	_____
		_____
_____	First Athletics	_____
		_____
_____	Normal Athletics	_____
		_____

Timeline Guide for Planning Your THR or Resurf

Event	Average Duration
Book Hospital	2–4 weeks prior to admission
Pre-Donation of Blood	3–5 days (optimal) prior to admission
Hospital Stay	2–5 days (can be more if medical condition pre- or post-op necessitates.)
Staple or Stitch Removal	2–3 Weeks post-op. This is done by visiting a nurse or MD
Home Aide	4–6 weeks
Supervised Physical Therapy	4–8 weeks (see insurance coverage)
First Post-Op Surgeon Visit	2–3 weeks after discharge
On Crutches	6–12 weeks
Return to Work	Your call (suggest 8 weeks, if you can use crutches and work at a sedentary position)
Use Public Transportation	6–8 weeks
Resume Sex Life	Your call (with position and activity precautions)
Drive Your Own Car	16–18 weeks
Need Rental Equipment	16–20 weeks
Return to Gym Workouts	6–8 weeks (Crossover with P.T. program and *modify* workout to avoid risk of hip dislocation; over-straining thigh, buttock, and calf muscles)
Stand in Line for Theaters, Restaurants, etc.	6–8 months
Use of Wheelchair in Airport	6–12 months

Planning for Your Discharge

Preparation is the key to making a smooth transition from the hospital to your home. Review the checklist below and talk to your doctor, discharge planner, or nurse about your questions or concerns. During your stay in the hospital the staff will work with you to plan for your discharge. For any questions below that you answer "No" to, check with hospital staff for further assistance.

Getting Ready to Go Home

Transportation

1. Is there someone to pick you up and take you home from the hospital?..........................❑ Yes   ❑ No

_____

_____

Name_____   Telephone_____
Address_____

Medications

1. Are you able to get your prescriptions filled when you leave the hospital? ....❑ Yes   ❑ No
2. Do you know what each prescription drug does?..❑ Yes   ❑ No
3. Do you know how and when to take them and the side effects?.....................................❑ Yes   ❑ No

_____

_____

Medical Supplies

1. Do you need to purchase medical equipment (like a walkerette, etc.)?...................................❑ Yes   ❑ No

_____

_____

Follow-Up Appointment

1. Did you schedule your follow-up appointments or tests? .... ❑ Yes   ❑ No
2. Do you know the time and location of your appointment? And the doctor's name? .... ❑ Yes   ❑ No
3. Will you have transportation to the appointment? .... ❑ Yes   ❑ No

_____

_____

Name_____ Telephone_____
Address_____

Home Maintenance

1. Will you need physical aids in the home, such as a bathroom grab bars? .... ❑ Yes   ❑ No
2. Do you feel you need extra assistance?
   a.   Changing bandage.................................. ❑ Yes   ❑ No
   b.   Bathing, dressing, using the bathroom ....❑ Yes   ❑ No
   c.   Preparing foods and running errands......❑ Yes   ❑ No

_____

_____

Name_____ Telephone_____
Address_____

Ongoing Treatment

1. Are you ready to help manage your condition at home? .... ❑ Yes   ❑ No
2. Should you do any special exercises? .... ❑ Yes   ❑ No
3. Do you need any home health services? .... ❑ Yes   ❑ No
   What type?_____
   How often? _____
4. Does your insurance cover home health services ordered by your doctor? .... ❑ Yes   ❑ No

_____

_____

Follow-up Appointment with Doctor

When did you do the following?	Weeks Post-Operative				
	3	6	8	10	12
Lie in bed on either side, including your operated hip.	■	■	❏	❏	❏
Lie in bed without using a pillow between your legs.	❏	❏	❏	❏	❏
How long to use the walker or crutches.	❏	❏	❏	❏	❏
Stop wearing graduated compression (white elastic) socks.	❏	❏	❏	❏	❏
Put on shoes and socks without long shoe horn.	■	■	❏	❏	❏
Bend to the floor.	■	■	■	■	❏
Take a bath.	■	❏	❏	❏	❏
Discontinue elevated toilet seat.	■	■	■	■	■
Drive a car.	■	❏	❏	❏	❏
Increase leisure activities (golfing, tennis, etc.).	■	■	■	■	■
Swelling went down.	■	❏	❏	❏	❏
Resume sexual activities.	■	❏	❏	❏	❏

Note: A black box (■) indicates you should not attempt.

Posthab Exercise Log

The post rehab process after total hip replacement occurs early in the post-operative period—actually within the first 6 to 8 weeks. Most patients start physical therapy the day after surgery to help regain and improve strength around the operative hip.

Post surgery, the goal of your exercise program should be to gradually restore normal hip motion and strength. Your orthopedic surgeon and physical therapist may recommend exercise for 20 to 30 minutes 2 or 3 times a day during early recovery. Do your best. Again, if you feel pain, speak up immediately.

Remember, you have just had major surgery—everything is not going to feel the same. The journey your muscles have endured through the operation leaves them tight and potentially sore. Therefore, start small, stretch first, and gradually grow from there with all levels of your exercise program.

Ankle Rotations (page 122)

Reps	Mon.	Tue.	Wed.	Thu.	Fri.	Sat.	Sun.
Week 1							
Week 2							
Week 3							
Week 4							

Bed-Supported Knee Bends (page 122)

Reps	Mon.	Tue.	Wed.	Thu.	Fri.	Sat.	Sun.
Week 1							
Week 2							
Week 3							
Week 4							

Buttock Contractions (page 122)

Reps	Mon.	Tue.	Wed.	Thu.	Fri.	Sat.	Sun.
Week 1							
Week 2							
Week 3							
Week 4							

Hip Abductor Exercise (page 123)

Reps	Mon.	Tue.	Wed.	Thu.	Fri.	Sat.	Sun.
Week 1							
Week 2							
Week 3							
Week 4							

Standing Knee Raises (page 123)

Reps	Mon.	Tue.	Wed.	Thu.	Fri.	Sat.	Sun.
Week 1							
Week 2							
Week 3							
Week 4							

Standing Hip Extensions (page 124)

Reps	Mon.	Tue.	Wed.	Thu.	Fri.	Sat.	Sun.
Week 1							
Week 2							
Week 3							
Week 4							

Standing Hip Abduction (page 124)

Reps	Mon.	Tue.	Wed.	Thu.	Fri.	Sat.	Sun.
Week 1							
Week 2							
Week 3							
Week 4							

"Step on Gas" Ankle Pumps (page 125)

Reps	Mon.	Tue.	Wed.	Thu.	Fri.	Sat.	Sun.
Week 1							
Week 2							
Week 3							
Week 4							

Resources

These agencies can give you and your caregiver more information about community services, like home-delivered meals and rides to appointments. Ask your social worker for more information about community services and support.

Area Agencies on Aging (AAAs)
AAAs assist adults age 60 and older and their caregivers. To find the AAA in your area, call The Eldercare Locator at 800-677-1116 weekdays from 9:00 am to 8:00 pm (EST) or visit www.eldercare.gov.

Aging and Disability Resource Centers (ADRCs)
ADRCs assist people of all incomes and ages. Forty-three states have ADRCs. To find out if your area is served by an ADRC, visit www.adrc-tae.org.

Centers for Independent Living (CILs)
CILs assist people with disabilities. A state-by-state directory of CILs can be found by visiting www.ilru.org/html/publications/directory/ index.html.

Medicare
For more information about the Medicare Program, call 800-MEDICARE (800-633-4227). TTY users should call 1-877-486-2048. You can also visit www.medicare.gov/LongTermCare/Static/ Counseling.asp.

State Technology Assistance Project
Their purpose is to improve the potential of people with disabilities to achieve their goals through the use of technology. They promote research, development, education, advocacy and provision of technology, and support the people engaged in these activities. Contact RESNA at 703-524-6686 or www.resna.org.

State Medicaid Agency
The State Medical Assistance (Medicaid) office provides information about Medicaid. To find your local office, visit www.nasmd.org/ links/links.asp. (Scroll halfway down the page to see a clickable map of the United States.) You can also call 800-MEDICARE.

Index

Mary Ellen Hecht, M.D., attended Columbia University for Pre-med and received her M.D. from the State University of New York (SUNY). She did her residency training in surgery and orthopedics at Long Island Jewish Hospital Center and was then awarded Clinical Instructor of Orthopedics at Mount Sinai School of Medicine.

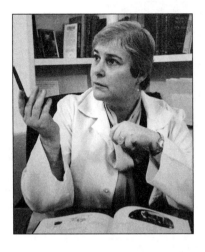

Dr. Hecht went on to become Assistant Chief of Orthopedics at Elmhurst Hospital, an affiliate of Mount Sinai School of Medicine, then into private practice until her retirement in 1998. Dr. Hecht divides her time between New Hope and Paris. Her personal passions include opera, theatre, and writing.

Also Available from Sunrise River Press

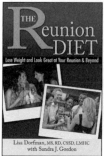

The Reunion Diet
Lose Weight and Look Great at Your Reunion and Beyond

by Lisa Dorfman with Sandra Gordon For millions of us, reunions offer a wake-up call and shore up weight-loss motivation. In *The Reunion Diet*, sports nutritionist Lisa Dorfman and health and nutrition writer Sandra J. Gordon show readers how to set specific weight-loss and other lifestyle goals and achieve them within the time allowed. At the core of the book is a diet plan calibrated by calorie levels according to how much time you have to lose weight before a reunion. Whether you've got 10, 20, 30 pounds or more to lose before your reunion, *The Reunion Diet* can help you look and feel great when mingling and reconnecting with those you may not have seen in decades. Softbound, 6 x 9 inches, 192 pages. **Item # SRP605**

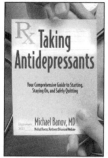

Taking Antidepressants
Your Comprehensive Guide to Starting, Staying On, and Safely Quitting

by Michael Banov, MD Antidepressants are the most commonly prescribed class of medications in this country. Yet, consumers have few available resources to educate them in a balanced fashion about starting and stopping antidepressants. Dr. Michael Banov walks the reader through a personalized process to help them make the right choice about starting antidepressants, staying on antidepressants, and stopping antidepressants. Readers will learn how antidepressant medications work, what they may experience while taking them, and will learn how to manage side effects or any residual or returning depression symptoms. Softbound, 6 x 9 inches, 304 pages. **Item # SRP606**

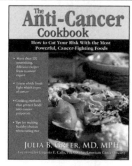

The Anti-Cancer Cookbook
How to Cut Your Risk with the Most Powerful, Cancer-Fighting Foods

by Dr. Julia Greer, MD, MPH Dr. Julia Greer explains what cancer is and how antioxidants work to prevent pre-cancerous mutations in your body's cells, and then describes which foods have been scientifically shown to help prevent which types of cancer. She then shares her collection of more than 220 scrumptious recipes for soups, sauces, main courses, vegetarian dishes, sandwiches, breads, desserts, and beverages, all loaded with nutritious ingredients chock-full of powerful antioxidants that may slash your risk of a broad range of cancer types. Softbound, 7.5 x 9 inches, 224 pages. **Item # SRP149**

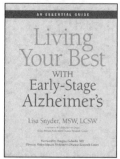

Living Your Best With Early-Stage Alzheimer's
An Essential Guide

by Lisa Snyder, MSW, LCSW Recent medical advances have made it possible to diagnose Alzheimer's when symptoms are only mild. New drugs are under investigation to help slow progression of the disease, and there is hope on the horizon for more effective treatments to keep the disease at bay. Today, when a person is diagnosed with Alzheimer's, they may have many years ahead with only mild symptoms. The result is that a growing number of people with early-stage Alzheimer's are seeking information about how to cope effectively with the disease. This book is a practical guide on effectively managing symptoms, finding meaningful activity, planning for the future, strategies for easier communication, participating in research and clinical trials, and much more. Numerous testimonials from people with Alzheimer's throughout the book give authenticity to the book content and provide practical suggestions as well as illuminating and insightful commentary. Softboubnd, 7 x 9 inches, 288 pages. **Item # SRP603**

www.sunriseriverpress.com or 1-800-895-4585